AAOS
Symposium on
The foot and leg
in running sports

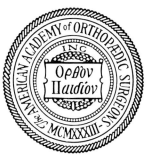

American Academy
of Orthopaedic Surgeons

Symposium on

The foot and leg in running sports

Coronado, California
September, 1980

Edited by

Robert P. Mack, M.D.
Attending Orthopaedic Surgeon,
St. Joseph's Hospital and Children's Hospital;
Orthopaedic Surgeon, Denver Sports Medicine Clinic,
Denver, Colorado

with 118 *illustrations*

The C. V. Mosby Company

ST. LOUIS • TORONTO • LONDON   1982

MOSBY

A TRADITION OF PUBLISHING EXCELLENCE

Editor: Eugenia A. Klein
Assistant editors: Kathryn H. Falk, Jean F. Carey
Manuscript editor: Patricia Tannian
Book design: Staff
Production: Barbara Merritt, Judith Bamert

Printed in the United States of America

The C.V. Mosby Company
11830 Westline Industrial Drive, St. Louis, Missouri 63141

Library of Congress Cataloging in Publication Data

Symposium on the Foot and Leg in Running Sports
(1980 : Coronado, Calif.)
   Symposium on the Foot and Leg in Running Sports,
Coronado, California, September, 1980.

   At head of title: American Academy of Orthopaedic
Surgeons.
   Bibliography: p.
   Includes index.
   1. Foot—Wounds and injuries.   2. Leg—Wounds and
injuries.   3. Running—Physiological aspects.
4. Running—Accidents and injuries—Prevention.
I. Mack, Robert P.   II. American Academy of
Orthopaedic Surgeons.   III. Title. [DNLM:
1. Running—Congresses.   2. Athletic injuries—
Congresses.   QT 260 S991s   1980]
RD563.S96   1980   617'.58   82-8188
ISBN 0-8016-0054-5

C/CB/B   9   8   7   6   5   4   3   2   1   05/C/597

Contributors

William J. Bowerman, Ph.D.

Professor Emeritus of Physical Education, University of Oregon; Track Coach Emeritus, 1972 United States Olympic Team, Eugene, Oregon

Peter R. Cavanagh, Ph.D.

Professor of Biomechanics, The Pennsylvania State University; Sports Science Advisor to Puma, University Park, Pennsylvania

Kenneth Cooper, M.D., M.P.H.

President and Founder, The Aerobics Center and the Institute for Aerobics Research; Author, *Aerobics; The New Aerobics; The Aerobics Way;* Co-author, *Aerobics for Women,* Dallas, Texas

David Drez, Jr., M.D.

Clinical Professor of Orthopaedics, Louisiana State University School of Medicine, New Orleans, Louisiana; Team Physician, McNeese State University, Lake Charles, Louisiana

Ejnar Eriksson, M.D.

Head, Section of Trauma, Department of Surgery, Karolinska Hospital, Stockholm, Sweden

Tom Häggmark, M.D.

Assistant Professor of Surgery, Department of Surgery, Karolinska Hospital, Stockholm, Sweden

Alan Hargens, Ph.D.

Associate Professor of Surgery, Division of Orthopaedics, Veterans Administration Hospital, San Diego, California

Douglas W. Jackson, M.D.

Director of Sports Medicine Clinic, Memorial Hospital Medical Center of Long Beach; Associate Clinical Professor of Surgery, University of Irvine, Long Beach, California

Robert E. Leach, M.D.

Professor and Chairman, Department of Orthopaedics, Boston University; Orthopaedic Consultant to Boston University and Northeastern University Athletic Teams, Boston, Massachusetts

Rolf Ljungqvist, M.D.

Assistant Professor of Orthopaedic Surgery, Serafimerlasarettet, Stockholm, Sweden

Roger A. Mann, M.D.

Associate Clinical Professor of Orthopaedic Surgery, University of California–San Francisco; Clinical Director of Gait Analysis Laboratory, Shriner's Hospital, San Francisco, California

Scott Mubarak, M.D.

Assistant Professor of Surgery, Division of Orthopaedics and Rehabilitation, University of California–San Diego, University Hospital, San Diego, California

Bruce C. Ogilvie, Ph.D.

Professor Emeritus, Department of Psychology, San Jose State University; Fellow, American College of Sports Medicine, San Jose, California

Allan N. Sutker, M.D.

Orthopedist, Plano Orthopedic and Sports Medicine Clinic, Plano, Texas

Alan M. Strizak, M.D.

Assistant Professor of Surgery, Chief of Sports Medicine, Division of Orthopedic Surgery, Harbor-UCLA Medical Center, Torrance, California

Dennis E. Vixie, C.O.

Director, Eugene Orthotic and Prosthetic Center; Member, American Academy of Orthotists and Prosthetists; Member, American Board for Certification in Orthotics and Prosthetics; Consultant, Nike Shoe Corporation, Eugene, Oregon

Richard Wallensten, M.D.

Department of Orthopaedic Surgery, Karolinska Hospital, Stockholm, Sweden

John F. Waller, Jr., M.D., P.C.

Chief, Foot and Ankle Service, Lenox Hill Hospital; Adjunct, Orthopaedic Department, Lenox Hill Hospital, New York, New York

Preface

Americans have recognized the importance of personal physical fitness, and millions have sought to improve their level of fitness by turning to running. As people of all ages have begun participating in running sports, many new and different medical problems have been presented to physicians. Physicians who have expressed an interest in runners' medical problems have been frustrated by the runner as a patient. Even more frustrating has been the lack of knowledge, data, and tools to help physicians understand and deal with runners' medical problems. The objective of this text is to provide a reference for physicians in treating these problems.

The American Academy of Orthopaedic Surgeons provided a forum for experts in the physiology of running and overuse syndromes in Coronado, California, on September 22-25, 1980. Two hundred fifty orthopaedic surgeons met to learn about running and its related medical problems. The kinetics and biomechanics of running and the relationship of the foot, shoe, and ground were discussed. Basic exercise physiology principles were presented and then applied as participants were tested on a treadmill. The multiple medical problems of the lower extremity and spine were reviewed with an emphasis on prevention, early recognition, proper treatment, and rehabilitation.

The importance of this meeting should be emphasized. It represents an attempt by orthopaedic surgeons to educate themselves concerning a new group of sports medicine problems that usually require nonoperative treatment. Much of the material presented at the meeting is included in this text.

As chairman of this course, I wish to thank the authors for their efforts and scientific data.

Robert P. Mack, M.D.

Contents

AAOS
Symposium on
The foot and leg in running sports

1. Biomechanics of running

Roger A. Mann

To understand the biomechanics of running, one must fully appreciate the biomechanics of walking, since the same basic mechanisms are functioning in the lower extremity and foot in both gaits. Two changes occur in the running gait: the increased magnitude of the vertical forces to two to three times body weight and the progressive shortening of the stance phase from 0.6 second to about 0.2 second. Both of these changes are affected greatly by the individual's running speed and running style. A good working knowledge of biomechanics of the lower extremities during running is extremely important in evaluating the various types of problems seen in the runner. An understanding of normal biomechanics may make it possible to identify the abnormal biomechanics present during running so that treatment can be on a firm scientific basis rather than on an empirical basis. The more precisely we can make a biomechanical diagnosis, the more precisely we can direct our treatment to achieve a satisfactory result.

The study of running includes many factors that do not apply to average, everyday walking. These include the speed of running, such as recreational jogging versus world-class sprinting, whether significant acceleration and deceleration are occurring during running, and the length of time that the activity is being carried out, for example, long-distance training versus sprint training. This discussion is largely confined to steady-state running of distances greater than 1 mile.

GAIT CYCLE

The gait cycle is the basic reference in the description of gait, making it possible to compare walking, jogging, and running very easily. The normal walking cycle begins with heel strike and ends with heel strike of the same foot. Therefore there are two steps in each gait cycle. In the case of a runner who is striking the ground on his toes, the gait cycle is from toe strike to toe strike.

The gait cycle is divided into the periods of stance phase and swing phase. In walking the stance phase consists of approximately 60% of the gait cycle and the swing phase of 40%. During the stance phase two periods of double limb support occur, the first one from 0% to 12% of the cycle and the second from 50% to 62%. Between these two periods of double limb support is a period of single limb support

1

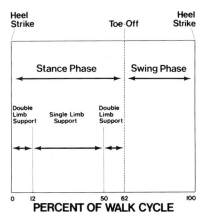

Fig. 1-1. Phases of walking cycle.

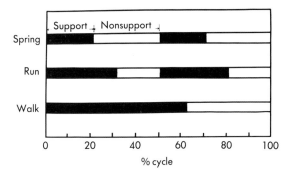

Fig. 1-2. Support or stance phase is in black and nonsupport or swing phase is in white. As speed of gait increases, period of support decreases and period of nonsupport increases.

that occupies approximately 35% of the walking cycle. One foot is always on the ground throughout the walking cycle (Fig. 1-1).

As the speed of gait increases, the period of stance phase progressively decreases and the period of swing phase increases (Fig. 1-2). There also occurs a float phase or period of nonsupport during which both feet are off the ground. Fig. 1-3 is a chart depicting walking, jogging, and running in real time, so that one can appreciate the overall decrease in the cycle time. The walker is moving at a comfortable walking speed of 120 steps per minute, and his total cycle time is 1 second. The jogger is proceeding at a rate of approximately 6 miles per hour, and his cycle time is 0.7 second. The runner is proceeding at approximately 12 miles per hour, and his cycle time is decreased to 0.6 second. However, the stance phase has decreased from 0.62 to 0.2 second. This marked decrease in the stance phase is one

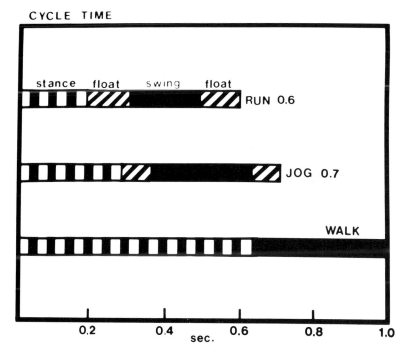

CYCLE TIME

Fig. 1-3. As speed of gait increases, there is period of time in which both feet are off the ground. This period is known as the float phase. As speed of gait increases, length of stance phase decreases and period of float phase increases. (From Bateman, J.E., and Trott, A.: The foot and ankle, © 1980 by Thieme-Stratton, Inc., New York.)

of the basic causes of injury in runners, since all the events—shock absorption, deceleration, transverse plane motion, foot stabilization, and acceleration—occur in approximately one third of the time that they occur in walkers. The angular velocity must likewise be increased to accommodate this rapid change in the cycle. Furthermore, the events of this shortened cycle time are repeated for many hours of training. For this reason any significant abnormality in the biomechanical system may be manifest in the form of a running injury in the lower extremity.

GROUND REACTION FORCE DURING GAIT

In concurrence with Newton's third law, which states that for every action there is an equal and opposite reaction, forces exerted by the body during gait can be measured by the use of a force plate. The forces presented in this discussion are the vertical, fore and aft shear, medial and lateral shear, and torque. Generally speaking, the ground reaction to walking is an extremely reproducible measurement, whereas during running and jogging there is much more variability from step to step. As the speed of gait increases, the ground reaction increases, and conversely, the slower one walks, the less the ground reaction.

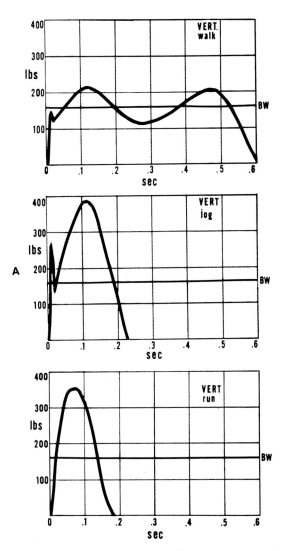

Fig. 1-4. Comparison of force plate analysis for walking, running, and jogging. **A,** Vertical force. (**A** through **D** from Bateman, J.E., and Trott, A.: The foot and ankle, © 1980 by Thieme-Stratton, Inc., New York.)

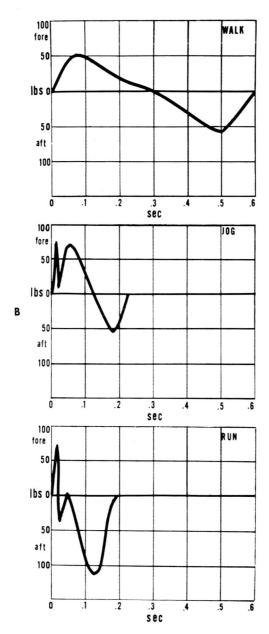

Fig. 1-4, cont'd. **B,** Fore and aft shear.
Continued.

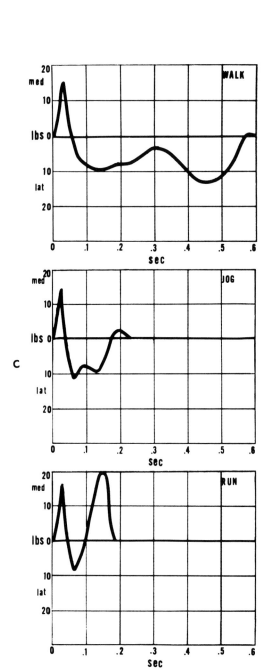

Fig. 1-4, cont'd. C, Medial lateral shear.

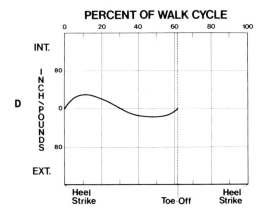

Fig. 1-4, cont'd. **D,** Force plate analysis of torque during walking.

The vertical force plate data in Fig. 1-4, *A,* demonstrate a marked increase in the initial spike, which represents the initial impact of the foot against the ground. During walking this rarely exceeds 70% to 80% of the body weight. During jogging it increases to almost twice body weight. The second peak in the vertical force increases from 110% to 115% of body weight during walking to approximately 275% during jogging and running. The twin peaks that are present during walking are not present during running, probably because only one foot is on the ground at a time during the running gait, whereas there are periods of double limb support during walking. The inclination of the curves is increased greatly in running because of the rapid loading and unloading of the foot.

The overall configuration of the fore and aft shear curves is essentially the same for walking and running, but the magnitude increases somewhat with running (Fig. 1-4, *B*).

The medial and lateral shear curves demonstrate the same basic pattern during walking and running. As the foot strikes the ground, the force is always driven in a medial direction or toward the midline, following which the leg exerts a force in a lateral direction. In running there seems to be a second period of medial shear that I am unable to explain at this time (Fig 1-4, *C*).

Torque occurs in response to transverse rotation in the lower extremity during gait (Fig. 1-4, *D*). The only torque measurement presented here is for walking, in which an internal torque at the time of ground contact is followed by a progressive external torque until the time of toe-off. This torque also occurs during running but has not yet been adequately quantitated. The torque measurement correlates well with the transverse rotation in the lower extremity, as demonstrated in Fig. 1-5. Progressive internal rotation occurs in the pelvis, femur, and tibia at the time of initial ground contact and reaches a peak at approximately 15% to 20% of the gait cycle, after which progressive external rotation proceeds until the time of toe-off.

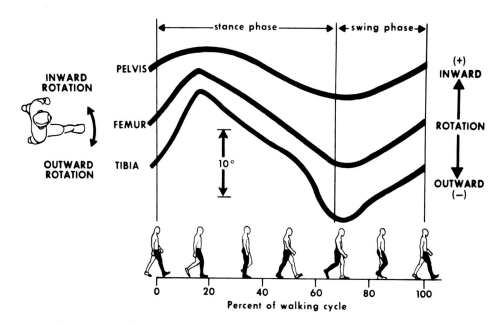

Fig. 1-5. Transverse plane rotation of pelvis, femur, and tibia. Maximum internal rotation is achieved by approximately 15% of walking cycle, and maximum external rotation occurs at time of toe-off. (From Mann, R.A.: Biomechanics of the foot. In American Academy of Orthopaedic Surgeons: Atlas of orthotics, St. Louis, 1975, The C.V. Mosby Co.)

ANGULAR ROTATION OF THE LOWER EXTREMITY

During normal locomotion, rotation is occurring in the sagittal, frontal, and transverse planes. This motion in all three planes during walking has been well documented and is quite consistent from person to person.[8,13,14] As the speed of gait increases, however, measurement of rotation in the transverse plane becomes much more difficult. Qualitative analysis of high-speed films showing gait demonstrates that the direction of the magnitude of transverse rotation is apparently unchanged from walking, but the quantitation of this data is thus far unreliable. Sagittal and frontal plane motion, however, is well documented and is presented in Fig. 1-6.

In reviewing the sagittal plane motion with increasing speed of gait, it becomes apparent that the total range of motion in the hip, knee, and ankle is increasing in magnitude but the period of time in which it is occurring is decreasing. As a result of this, the curve becomes steep as the speed of gait increases (Fig. 1-7).

The configuration and magnitude of the hip abduction-adduction pattern remain essentially the same during walking and running.

The transverse plane rotation in walking is presented in Fig. 1-5. As mentioned previously, the direction of the rotation remains essentially the same for running as for walking, with internal rotation occurring at the time of initial ground contact and external rotation at the time of toe-off. The magnitude seems to be approxi-

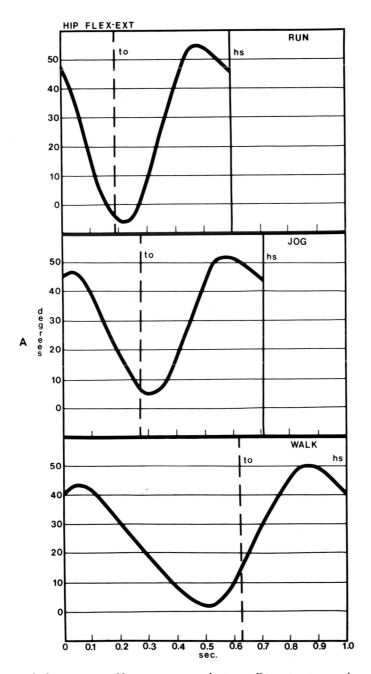

Fig. 1-6. Sagittal plane motion of lower extremity during walking, jogging, and running. *to,* Toe-off; *hs,* heel strike. **A,** Hip joint. *Continued.*

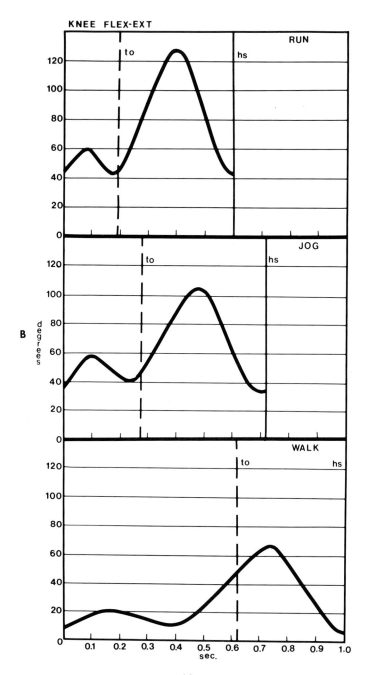

Fig. 1-6, cont'd. **B,** Knee joint.

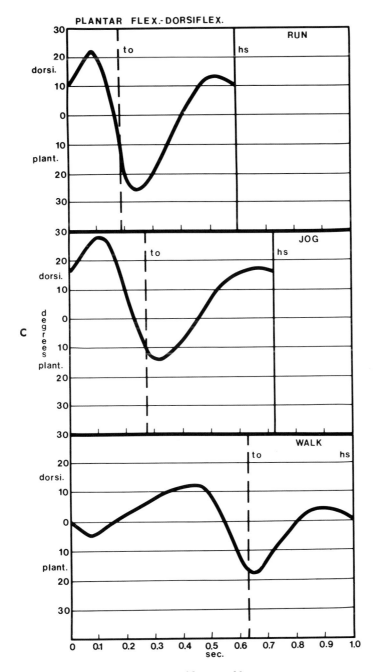

Fig. 1-6, cont'd. C, Ankle joint.

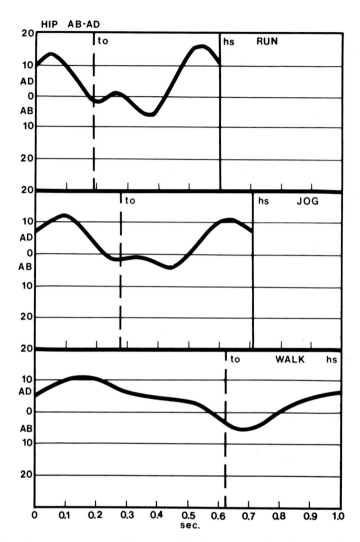

Fig. 1-7. Frontal plane motion of hip joint (hip abduction and adduction) during walking, jogging, and running. *to,* Toe-off; *hs,* heel strike.

mately the same for running as for walking. It must be emphasized, however, that this transverse plane rotation is occurring over a period of about 0.2 second during running, as compared to 0.6 second during walking. Excessive transverse plane rotation may cause clinical problems in the hip, knee, ankle, or subtalar joints.

ELECTROMYOGRAPHY OF THE LOWER EXTREMITIES

The term "phasic activity of muscle" refers to the period during the gait cycle in which there is electrical activity within the muscle. During the period of muscle activity the muscle may be undergoing a concentric (shortening) contraction or an eccentric (lengthening) contraction. Some muscles, such as the anterior compart-

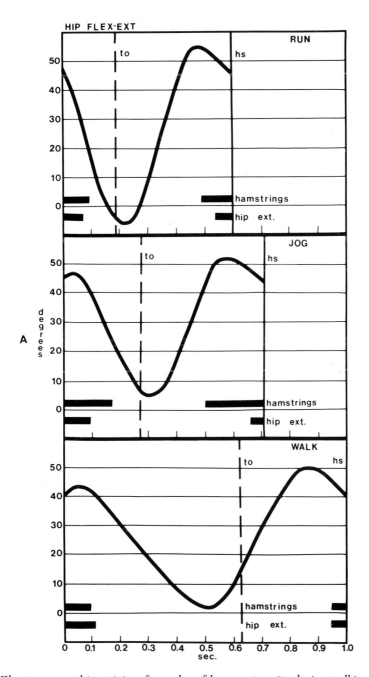

Fig. 1-8. Electromyographic activity of muscles of lower extremity during walking, jogging, and running in relation to range of motion of joint. *to,* Toe-off; *hs,* heel strike. **A,** Hip joint. (**A** and **B** from Bateman, J.E., and Trott, A.: The foot and ankle, © 1980 by Thieme-Stratton, Inc., New York.) *Continued.*

Fig. 1-8, cont'd. B, Knee joint.

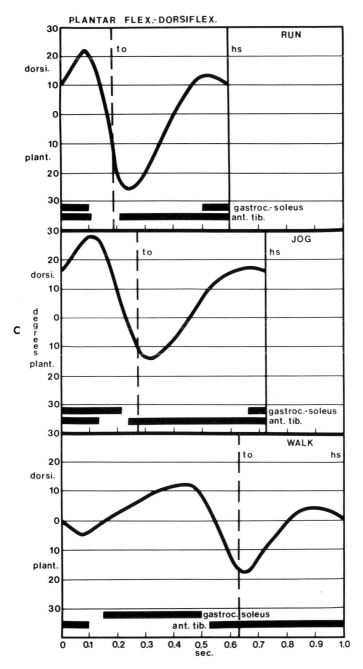

Fig. 1-8, cont'd. **C,** Ankle joint.

Continued.

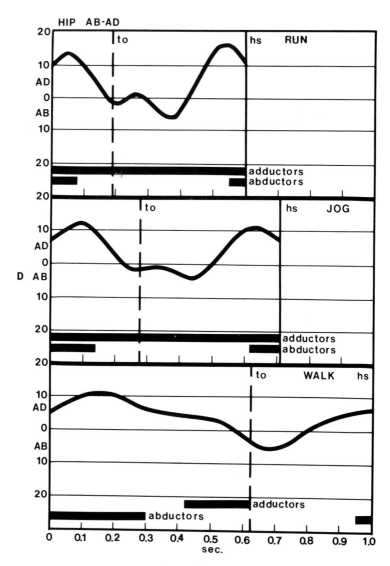

Fig. 1-8, cont'd. **D,** Hip joint.

ment muscles of the leg, undergo a concentric contraction at the beginning of phasic activity and an eccentric contraction at the end. Conversely, some muscles, such as those of the posterior calf, undergo an eccentric contraction initially, followed by a concentric contraction. In studying the phasic activity of the muscles in the lower extremity, our laboratory has consistently noted that these muscles function as groups rather than individually. We have placed electrodes on the muscles that comprise the quadriceps group and on the hamstrings and have noted no significant variation in the individual muscles within these groups. The same has been noted for the anterior calf muscles and the superficial muscles of the posterior calf and lateral compartment. Although we do not have adequate information on the deep muscles of the posterior calf, I believe these muscles also work as a functional unit, and they are considered as such in presenting this data.

As the speed of gait increases, the total time of muscle activity in the lower extremity increases somewhat when measured in real time but increases greatly as a percentage of the gait cycle. The phasic activity of certain muscle groups of the lower extremity in relation to the range of motion of the joints is presented in Fig. 1-8.

BIOMECHANICAL MECHANISMS OF THE LOWER LIMB

The biomechanical events occurring in the lower limb at the time of initial ground contact include shock absorption, joint stabilization of the hip, knee, and ankle, and foot flexibility. As mentioned previously, the magnitude of these events increases many fold as the speed of gait increases. The shock absorption occurs through the flexion present in the hip and knee joints, the dorsiflexion at the ankle joint, and the eversion at the subtalar joint. The joint stability is brought about by activity in the muscle groups crossing the hip, knee, and ankle joints, which are electrically active at the time of initial ground contact. (The hip flexors, however, are not functional.) The foot flexibility results from eversion of the subtalar joint, which produces a degree of relaxation of the midtarsal joints and subsequent relaxation of the other stabilization mechanisms within the arch of the foot. Once the foot has been fully loaded and the center of gravity has passed in front of the base of support, progressive stabilization occurs within the foot to produce a rigid structure for the support and propulsive portions of the stance phase.

The stabilization mechanism involves the transverse rotation occurring in the lower extremity. There is internal rotation in the lower limb at the time of initial ground contact, followed by progressive external rotation after the foot has been fully loaded. This external rotation is brought about by several mechanisms. The first is the forward motion of the contralateral pelvis. As the contralateral pelvis is being brought forward, in part by the rapidly flexing thigh, it functions as a crank to help impart external rotation to the stance limb. This external rotation seems to occur because of the firm attachment of the pelvis to the stance leg femur by the electrically active adductor muscles. The external rotation force, which is probably sizeable considering the degree of leverage involved in the system, is passed across the knee and ankle joints and is translated by the subtalar joint to the arch of the foot. The subtalar joint, which acts as an oblique hinge aligned at approximately 45 degrees to the horizontal and deviating from medial to lateral 16 degrees in relation to the long axis of the foot, translates the transverse rotation of the lower extremity into inversion and eversion of the calcaneus (Fig. 1-9).[2,10,15] This rotation in the subtalar joint essentially controls the subsequent stability of the forefoot through its control of the transverse tarsal joint and therefore affects the stability of the longitudinal arch of the foot. The function of the transverse tarsal joint, which is made up of the talonavicular and calcaneocuboid joints, is such that inversion of the

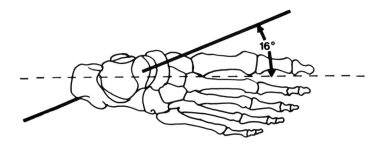

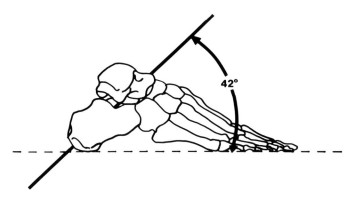

Fig. 1-9. Axis of subtalar joint.

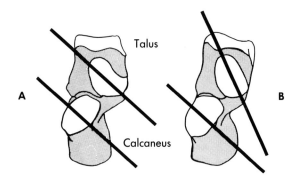

Talus

Calcaneus

Fig. 1-10. Axes of transverse tarsal joint. **A,** When calcaneus is in eversion, conjoint axes between talonavicular and calcaneocuboid joints are parallel to one another so that increased motion occurs in transverse tarsal joint. **B,** When calcaneus is in inversion, axes are no longer parallel and there are decreased motion and increased stability of transverse tarsal joint.

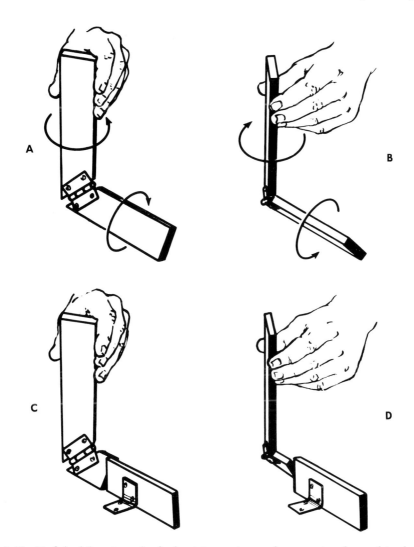

Fig. 1-11. Model of function of subtalar joint as it translates motion from tibia above to calcaneus below. **A,** Action of mitered hinge demonstrates translation of rotation across 45-degree hinge. This is analogous to subtalar joint. Inward rotation of upper stick causes outward rotation of lower stick. This is analogous to inward rotation of tibia, producing eversion of calcaneus. **B,** Outward rotation of tibia produces inward rotation of calcaneus. **C** and **D,** Addition of pivot between two segments of mechanism presents same analogy as above but with addition of transverse tarsal joint. This is depicted by pivot point beyond 45-degree hinge working against distal segment, which is fixed to the ground. This distal segment represents forefoot, which is firmly planted on the ground. Inward rotation of tibia, which produces eversion of calcaneous, obviously has effect on transverse tarsal joint. See text for further explanation. (From Inman, V.T., and Mann, R.A.: Biomechanics of the foot and ankle. In Mann, R.A., editor: Duvries' surgery of the foot, ed. 4, St. Louis, 1978, The C.V. Mosby Co.)

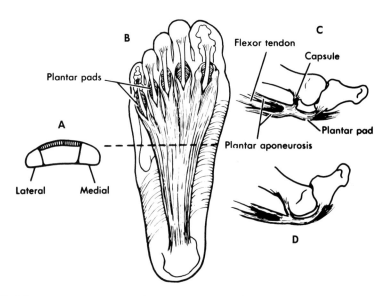

Fig. 1-12. Plantar aponeurosis. **A,** Cross-section. **B,** Plantar aponeurosis divides as it proceeds distally to allow flexor tendons to pass through aponeurosis. **C,** Plantar aponeurosis combines with joint capsule to form plantar pad of metatarsophalangeal joint. **D,** Dorsiflexion of toes forces metatarsal head into plantar flexion and brings plantar pad over head of metatarsal. (From Mann, R., and Inman, V.T.: Structure and function. In Mann, R.A., editor: Duvries' surgery of·the foot, ed. 4, St. Louis, 1978, The C.V. Mosby Co.)

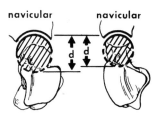

Fig. 1-13. Relationship of head of talus to navicular. Left superior and right lateral views show differing diameter of head of talus.

calcaneus brings about increased stability of the transverse tarsal joint and eversion of the subtalar joint brings about decreased stability of the transverse tarsal joint (Figs. 1-10 and 1-11).[3]

Other mechanisms within the foot itself help to bring about stability in the last half of the stance phase. The plantar aponeurosis arises from the tubercle of the calcaneus and passes forward to insert into the base of the proximal phalanges. As the proximal phalanx is dorsiflexed onto the metatarsal head near the time of toe-off, the plantar aponeurosis is wrapped around the metatarsal head and depresses

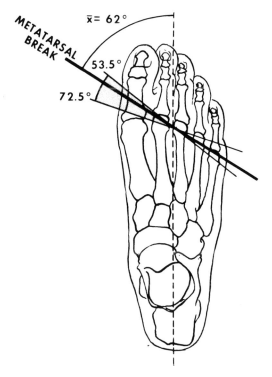

Fig. 1-14. Variation in angulation of metatarsal break. (From Mann, R.A.: Biomechanics of the foot. In American Academy of Orthopaedic Surgeons: Atlas of orthotics, St. Louis, 1975, The C.V. Mosby Co.; redrawn from Inman, R.E., and Inman, V.T.: Anthropometric studies of the human foot and ankle, Bull. Prosthet. Res. **10:**11, 1969.)

it.[4] Through this mechanism the longitudinal arch is elevated without the use of muscle force per se (Fig. 1-12). At the same time that the plantar aponeurosis is functioning, the intrinsic muscles of the foot are active[9]; these help to stabilize the longitudinal arch in much the same way as does the plantar aponeurosis.

The shape of the talonavicular joint is such that as force is applied across it, its stability is increased. If we look at the head of the talus in the anterior posterior plane and circumscribe a circle along the articular surface and then do the same in the lateral plane, we create circles of different diameters. Thus as the talonavicular joint is loaded, increasing stability is brought about by the seating of the convex head of the talus into the concave navicular (Fig. 1-13).

The metatarsal break is an axis represented by an oblique line passing roughly across the metatarsal heads.[5,7] It can be observed on one's shoe by looking at the oblique crease in the top of the shoe material over the metatarsophalangeal joints. The importance of the metatarsal break is that, as the toes are forced into dorsiflexion, the obliquely placed axis helps to bring about external rotation of the stance leg (Fig. 1-14).

MUSCLE FUNCTION DURING RUNNING
Hip joint

The muscle groups of the hip joint that have been studied at our Gait Analysis Laboratory at the Shriners' Hospital in San Francisco are the gluteus maximus, hamstrings, hip abductors, and hip adductors. During walking the gluteus maximus is active from the end of swing phase until the foot is flat on the ground at approximately 10% of the walking cycle. The hamstring muscles demonstrate a similar period of activity. These two muscle groups probably function to decelerate the swinging thigh and initiate extension of the hip joint. When these muscles cease to function, only a few degrees of extension of the joint has occurred. During jogging and running the gluteus maximus continues to have late swing phase activity, and the period of activity during the stance phase increases to approximately 30% of stance during jogging and nearly 50% during running. Rapid hip extension occurs during the stance phase and muscle activity, and the gluteus maximus probably plays a role in bringing about this extension. Approximately 25% of the hip joint extension is brought about during jogging and slightly more extension during running while the gluteus maximus is functioning.

The hamstring muscles demonstrate a longer period of swing and stance phase activity during jogging and running. The hamstrings are active during the last 50% of the swing phase during jogging and the last 25% of the swing phase during running. The hamstrings are active for approximately 50% of the initial stance phase of running and jogging. They probably function synergistically with the gluteus maximus to bring about rapid hip joint extension during the running gait.

The hip abductors demonstrate essentially the same period of activity in all speeds of gait. The abductors become active late in the swing phase and remain active during approximately the first 50% of the stance phase. The abductors function to stabilize the stance leg hemipelvis at the time of initial ground contact, thereby preventing excessive sagging of the swing leg hemipelvis.[6]

During walking the hip adductors are active in the last third of the stance phase, whereas during jogging and running their period of activity seems to extend throughout the entire stance and swing phases. However, great variability exists in the function of the hip adductor muscles from subject to subject, and a larger group of runners must be studied before we can definitely state the phasic activity of these muscles.

Knee joint

During walking the quadriceps muscles become active late in the swing phase and remain active during the stance phase until the initial period of knee flexion has been completed and extension of the knee joint once again begins (15% of the gait cycle). The quadriceps group functions to stabilize the knee at the time of initial ground contact and during the ensuing period of initial flexion. During jogging, the same phasic activity is noted as during walking. During running, however, the period of quadriceps activity during the swing phase increases considerably, probably to help bring about knee extension, which passes through a much greater arc of motion than during walking. The stance phase activity, although consuming nearly 50% of the stance phase, in real time is briefer than during walking. As mentioned previously, we have placed electrodes on the various muscles comprising the quadriceps group and have found that the periods of electrical activity do not seem to vary significantly among them.

The hamstring muscles, which were included in the previous discussion of the hip joint, must also be considered when discussing the knee joint, since they cross behind the knee as they insert into the tibia. It is difficult to state with any assurance which joint is most affected by the hamstring muscles during their stance phase period of activity. It would appear, however, that since the knee joint is flexing during the early stance phase while the hamstrings are active, this muscle group probably helps to stabilize the knee joint at the time of initial ground contact and actively helps produce extension at the hip joint. The flexion at the knee joint during this period of hamstring activity seems to be brought about by the weight of the body against the knee, rather than by the hamstrings. During the late swing phase the hamstrings may function to modulate the speed of knee extension and probably help to initiate hip extension.

Ankle joint

Significant changes occur in the function of the muscle groups about the ankle joint as the speed of gait increases. During walking the anterior compartment muscles (anterior tibial, extensor hallucis longus, and extensor digitorum longus) become active late in the stance phase and remain active throughout the swing phase until the plantigrade position has been achieved following initial ground contact. These muscles undergo an eccentric or lengthening contraction at the end of the stance phase, a concentric or shortening contracture during the swing phase, and then another eccentric or lengthening contraction after initial ground contact until the foot is flat on the ground. During the late stance phase, before toe-off, they probably function to help stabilize the foot and ankle, after which they produce dorsiflexion at the ankle joint to provide adequate toe clearance during the swing phase and control the initial plantar flexion at the time of initial ground contact. As the speed of gait increases, the anterior compartment muscles continue to function in a similar way during the swing phase, but during the stance phase there is a distinct change in their activity. As pointed out previously, at the time of initial ground contact during running, dorsiflexion occurs at the ankle joint and the anterior compartment muscles undergo a concentric contraction. The anterior compartment muscles then remain active during approximately 50% of the stance phase and cease to function just after plantar flexion of the ankle joint begins. Possibly this muscle group functions both to provide stability to the ankle at the time of initial ground contact and to accelerate the tibia over the fixed foot; this would be a very efficient mechanism by which the body could accelerate its forward movement during running. The posterior calf muscle group, including the gastroc-soleus group and the peroneal muscles, appears to function as a unit. During walking this group is active in the midstance phase, when it resists the progressive dorsiflexion of the ankle joint through an eccentric or lengthening contraction.[11,12] After it initiates plantar flexion of the ankle joint, its activity ceases. During running, however, this muscle group becomes active late in the swing phase and remains active for approximately 70% of the stance phase. The late swing phase and initial stance phase activity probably provide stability to the ankle joint and control the forward movement of the tibia over the fixed foot. During this period the muscle group is undergoing an eccentric or lengthening contraction. After about 50% of plantar flexion has occurred, this muscle group becomes electrically silent, leaving the remainder of the plantar flexion to be brought about by more passive mechanisms that are not yet well understood. Some investigators estimate that the force at the ankle joint during initial ground contact is approximately 10 times body weight. With this amount of force being applied across a small surface area, the importance of the stabilizing function of the muscle groups that cross the ankle cannot be overestimated.

There is controversy regarding the amount of push-off accomplished by the posterior calf group during steady-state walking. Most investigators who have studied the posterior calf muscles believe that the main function of this group during walking is to restrain the forward movement of the tibia rather than to push the body forward (push-off). It appears that in steady-state running the posterior calf group has the same basic function. This, however, should not be confused with the push-off by the posterior calf group during the acceleration phase of running, as well as during sports that require rapid starting and stopping, such as squash, basketball, and racquetball.

EVENTS OF A COMPLETE RUNNING CYCLE

Up to this point most of the components of the gait cycle have been presented as individual entities. It is important to remember that during running many of these events occur simultaneously to produce a coordinated sequence of movements. This section describes the sequence of movements that occurs during each running cycle.

We begin with the body in space during the float phase of the cycle. The center of gravity of the body reaches its peak elevation during the float phase. The body maintains a forward lean throughout the entire running cycle. Before initial ground contact there is a reversal of hip flexion, rapid knee extension, and dorsiflexion at the ankle joint. These joint motions carried out in the terminal float phase prepare the body for the impact of initial ground contact. At the moment of initial ground contact an initial spike is noted on the vertical force curve, which is equivalent to approximately 150% to 200% of body weight, as well as a forward shear force equal to about 50% of body weight and a medial shear force equal to approximately 10% of body weight. As the foot comes in contact with the ground, rapid extension of the hip joint, rapid flexion of the knee, and further dorsiflexion of the ankle take place. This motion in the knee and ankle joints helps to absorb the impact of the body striking the ground. The other mechanism helping to absorb this impact is the controlled pronation of the foot. As the lower limb strikes the ground, internal rotation occurs throughout the limb, helping to bring about the eversion of the calcaneous and the subsequent unlocking of the transverse tarsal joint, which in turn produces flexibility within the foot. The accommodation by the foot to the ground provides the body with a firm platform from which to function. Adduction of the hip joint is also occurring at this time. All of these joint motions are under direct control of the muscles that cross the joints. At the time of initial ground contact, essentially all of the muscles crossing the hip, knee, and ankle joints are functioning to provide stability to the joints and to help absorb the impact of initial ground contact.

The absorption mechanism for the initial ground impact continues for approximately 50% of the stance phase, with progressive dorsiflexion of the ankle joint and flexion of the knee joint. During this period rapid hip extension of the stance limb occurs, probably as a result of the rapid flexion taking place in the swinging thigh. Once the swinging leg has passed the stance leg base of support and the center of gravity is once again in front of the stance foot, progressive external rotation occurs in the pelvis. This external rotation of the pelvis, which is initiated by the swinging leg hip, rotates the stance leg pelvis externally because of the firm attachment of the pelvis to the thigh by the electrically active adductor muscles. The external rotation is passed across the knee and ankle joints into the foot, causing progressive inversion of the calcaneus and subsequent stabilization of the transverse tarsal joint and longitudinal arch of the foot. As this stabilizing mechanism is occurring during the last half of the stance phase, progressive extension of the hip and knee joints and rapid plantar flexion of the ankle joint take place. It should be noted parenthetically that before the onset of extension of the knee joint and plantar flexion of the ankle joint, the center of gravity has reached its lowest point during the stance phase. The hip joint during this period is undergoing progressive abduction. The ground reaction at the time of midstance demonstrates a vertical force approximating 250% to 300% of body weight and an aft shear equal to approximately 60% of body weight. As the body proceeds into the last third of the stance phase, the muscles about the ankle, knee, and hip joints (except possibly the adductors) cease their electrical activity. This suggests that once the absorption of initial ground contact has been completed and the center of gravity has passed in front of the stance leg foot, the majority of the forward propulsion of the body is coming from the swinging leg and arm motion rather than from the stance limb. The forward motion seems to be brought about by a combination of factors, including the rapid movement of the tibia over the fixed foot, the action of the flexing hip and swinging thigh, and the motion in the arms.

As the body begins the float phase, stability of the foot is maximum and internal rotation of the lower limb begins. The only muscles functioning about the knee and ankle at this moment are in the anterior compartment. Rapid flexion of the hip joint under the control of the iliopsoas muscle begins, along with passive flexion of the knee and active dorsiflexion of the ankle under the control of the anterior compartment musculature. No forces are acting against the foot after it leaves the ground and throughout the swing phase. During the middle to latter part of the swing or float phase, active hip flexion has reached its peak, the passive flexion of the knee joint reaches a peak at midswing and rapid active extension begins, and rapid progressive dorsiflexion continues at the ankle joint. Rapid adduction takes place at the hip joint during the last half of the swing phase. As the terminal swing phase is reached, there is a reversal of the hip flexion, and extension begins along with continued extension of the knee joint and continued dorsiflexion of the ankle joint. During the last 25% of the swing phase the hip extensors and hamstrings, the quadriceps group about the knee, and the posterior calf group become electrically active, probably in preparation for the impact of initial ground contact.

PRONATION

At the time of initial ground contact, one mechanism by which the body helps to dissipate the force is pronation of the foot. Pronation is not an isolated movement of a single joint but rather a complex sequence of motions that occurs throughout the foot and ankle joint. It produces a flexible foot at the time of weight acceptance. The opposite of pronation is supination, which produces a fairly rigid foot at the time of toe-off. As an individual stands at rest, the foot is in a pronated position and is fairly flexible. Conversely, as the individual stands on tiptoe, the foot is supinated and moderately rigid. The pronation occurring at the time of initial ground contact is a passive event brought about when the body weight is loaded onto the foot through the talus and subsequently loaded onto the subtalar joint, which by virtue of its configuration collapses into a pronated, everted position. The constraints of this pronation are the shape of the individual joints of the subtalar joint complex, their ligamentous support, and to a lesser degree the supporting musculature. As pronation occurs, the eversion of the subtalar joint causes obligatory internal rotation in the tibia. The degree of motion of the subtalar joint during walking has been quantitated in a person with normal feet at approximately 6 to 8 degrees, whereas a person with flatfeet has 10 to 12 degrees of motion. Since the rotation in the leg depends in part on the degree of rotation in the subtalar joint, it follows that the greater the pronation or eversion, the greater the degree of rotation in the tibia. This rotation in the tibia is not an isolated event but is passed on to the knee and hip joints. Thus an individual with hyperpronation of the foot has increased transverse plane motion in the lower extremity, and this may cause a clinical problem. The opposite effect occurs in an individual with a cavus foot, since a cavus foot has decreased motion in the subtalar joint and therefore decreased rotation in the tibia and lower extremity. This lack of motion of the subtalar joint results in decreased ability of the foot to dissipate the force of initial ground contact. Therefore the forces tend to be concentrated in several areas on the plantar aspect of the foot, which may result in clinical symptoms.

During walking, although the forces on the foot exceed body weight at times, the total amount of repetitive stress does not begin to approach that observed in an individual in a running program. Besides their normal everyday walking, avid runners travel another 30 to 50 miles per week on their feet, which undergo greatly increased stress. When an individual who weighs 150 pounds walks for 1 mile with a step length of $2^{1}/_{2}$ feet, he takes approximately 2110 steps. Thus at initial ground contact, considering an impact of 80% of body weight, he absorbs a total of 253,440 pounds (127 tons) or $63^{1}/_{2}$ tons on each foot. If the same individual runs 1 mile taking a step of $4^{1}/_{2}$ feet, which would result in approximately 1175 steps, he absorbs at initial ground contact, considering an impact of 250% of body weight, a total of 440,275 pounds (220 tons) or 110 tons on each foot. These figures are for only 1 mile, and it is readily apparent that after a 10-mile run the amount of force dissipated by the foot is considerable. Any biomechanical abnormality could result in a significant concentration of stress, producing the various clinical problems associated with running.

Another factor to be considered when discussing energy absorption within the foot is the time interval during which the foot is on the ground. During normal walking at a rate of 120 steps per minute, each walking cycle (from heel strike to heel strike of the same foot) consumes 1 second. The stance portion of this cycle is approximately 60% or in real time 0.6 second. If a runner is proceeding at approximately 6 minutes per mile, the total cycle time is 0.6 second and the stance phase is approximately 0.2 second. By increasing speed the runner has decreased the time the foot is on the ground from 0.6 second (600 msec) to 0.2 second (200 msec). Therefore all the events occurring during the stance phase must occur three times faster as the speed of gait is increased. The period of time between initial ground contact and maximum pronation is 0.15 second or 150 msec during walking but 0.03 second or 30 msec during running. In a study by Cavanagh and co-workers[1] in which an estimate was made of the angular velocity of pronation, it was noted that although maximum pronation occurs in 30 msec in an individual running a 6-minute mile, the actual angular velocity of the subtalar joint reaches a maximum in 15 msec. This maximum velocity is probably explained by the fact that as the foot strikes the ground, the heel is in a slightly inverted position. At initial ground contact the calcaneus is rapidly brought out of this slightly inverted position by the rapid weight acceptance it is undergoing. The remainder of the weight acceptance and associated pronation are carried out at a slightly slower rate. Another interesting correlation is that the medial shear force reaches its peak after approximately 10 msec. This is probably accounted for at least in part by the adducted position of the thigh and the inverted position of the subtalar joint at the time of initial ground contact. Following this initial medial shear is a progressive lateral shear that reaches its peak in 30 msec. This probably corresponds to the time that maximum pronation of the foot has occurred.

EFFECT OF AN ORTHOTIC DEVICE ON HINDFOOT MOTION

As noted in the previous section, the amount of energy that must be absorbed by the body during running is significant, and the more miles an individual runs, the greater the energy absorption required. In a small percentage of runners an overuse syndrome develops as a result of the body's inability to cope with repetitive stress without developing signs of fatigue. Runners with the overuse syndrome tend to have a more pronated foot than that noted in the average population, but this problem also has occurred in some patients with a cavus foot. Other types of malalignment syndromes include genu varum and valgum, internal and external tibial torsion, and femoral anteversion and retroversion. These conditions often cause symptoms because of repeated stress on a certain part of the lower extremity or because of the runner's attempt to compensate for a physical abnormality.

Various orthotic devices have been fabricated for runners, including both the rigid acrylic type and the soft pliable type. The question that always arises is what, if anything, an orthotic device does for the foot from a biomechanical standpoint. Although several investigators have studied the effect of an orthotic on motion in the lower extremity, this question remains unanswered. Information regarding the transverse rotation of the lower extremity during running is technically extremely difficult to obtain. Likewise, measuring the motion of the subtalar joint during running presents many technical problems. Since measurements cannot be obtained, the subtle differences probably brought about by the use of an orthotic device cannot be quantitated, and not much more than an educated guess can be made about the effect of these devices.

By the use of high-speed photography in our laboratory, we have been able to obtain a qualitative idea of the motion occurring in the subtalar joint and the transverse rotation of the tibia. The motion in the subtalar joint during running is similar to that seen during walking except it occurs much more rapidly. The addition of a support to the medial side of the foot (medial arch support) brings about a decrease in the eversion of the calcaneus and the internal rotation of the tibia at the time of initial ground contact. The thicker the material used, the greater the decrease in pronation of the foot. In a study by Cavanagh and co-workers,[1] increasing thicknesses of felt were placed along the medial side of the foot, eventually reaching 9.5 mm of material. The runners demonstrated not only a decrease in the degree of pronation but also a marked decrease in the angular velocity by which the pronation occurred. In further studying these subjects with the use of a force plate, the investigators also demonstrated a significant change in the medial and lateral shear. The medial shear, which probably represents initial pronation of the foot, was decreased considerably in subjects using the medial support. It therefore appears that the use of an orthosis that provides medial support does play a role in the control of pronation by decreasing the total degree of eversion of the calcaneus and hence pronation at initial foot contact, as well secondarily controlling the transverse rotation imparted to the tibia. Altering this rotation of the tibia may correct the clinical symptoms affecting the knee and hip joints in some runners.

REFERENCES

1. Cavanagh, P.R., and others: An evaluation of the effect of orthotics on force distribution and rearfoot movement during running. Paper presented at the American Orthopaedics Society Sports Medicine Meeting, Lake Placid, New York, June 1978.
2. Close, J.R., and Inman, V.T.: The action of the subtalar joint, Univ. Calif. Prosthet. Devices Res. Rep. **11**:1, 1953.
3. Elftman, H.: The transverse tarsal joint and its control, Clin. Orthop. **16**:41, 1960.
4. Hicks, J.H.: The mechanics of the foot. II. The plantar aponeurosis and the arch, J. Anat. **88**:25, 1954.
5. Inman, R.E., and Inman, V.T.: Anthropometric studies of the human foot and ankle, Bull. Prosthet. Res. **10**:11, 1969.
6. Inman, V.T.: Functional aspects of the abductor muscles of the hip, J. Bone Joint Surg. **29A**:607, 1947.
7. Inman, V.T.: The joints of the ankle, Baltimore, 1976, The Williams & Wilkins Co.
8. Levens, A.D., Inman, V.T., and Blosser, J.A.: Transverse rotation of the segments of the lower extremity in locomotion, J. Bone Joint Surg. **30A**:859, 1948.
9. Mann, R.A., and Inman, V.T.: Phasic activity of the intrinsic muscles of the foot, J. Bone Joint Surg. **46A**:469, 1964.
10. Manter, J.T.: Movements of the subtalar and transverse tarsal joints, Anat. Rec. **80**:397, 1941.
11. Simon, S.R., and others: Role of the posterior calf muscles in normal gait, J. Bone Joint Surg. **60A**:465, 1978.
12. Sutherland, D.H.: An electromyographic study of the plantar flexors of the ankle in normal walking on the level, J. Bone Joint Surg. **48A**:66, 1966.
13. Sutherland, D.H., and Hagy, J.L.: Measurement of gait movements from motion picture films, J. Bone Joint Surg. **54A**:787, 1972.
14. University of California (Berkeley), Prosthetic Devices Research Project: Subcontractor's final report to the Committee on Artificial Limbs, National Research Council fundamental studies of human locomotion and other information relating to design of artificial limbs (in two volumes), Berkeley, Calif., 1947.
15. Wright, D.G., Desai, S.M., and Henderson, W.H.: Action of the subtalar and ankle-joint complex during the stance phase of walking, J. Bone Joint Surg. **46A**:361, 1964.

2. The shoe-ground interface in running

Peter R. Cavanagh

Events at the shoe-ground interface are difficult for the orthopaedic practitioner to evaluate on a routine basis. Although such relevant parameters as ranges of joint motion can be obtained with ease, there is some mystery about what goes on under the running shoe. The cause of the difficulty is that once the foot has reached a plantigrade position, the major events taking place there are invisible and cannot be determined without instrumentation. An example is a barefoot patient standing still with normal weight distribution under the left foot but with a small stone underneath the ball of the right foot. Obviously there are large pressures on the structures overlying the stone, but unless the patient is in pain, such an anomalous pressure distribution cannot be observed directly. A more realistic example is a patient with a plantar flexed first ray. The physician might suspect the patient is experiencing abnormally high forces under the first metatarsal head during ground contact in running, but there is no way to confirm this speculation through simple observation. Even the visible events such as the approach to the ground and the process of toeing off occur fast enough to deceive the eye.

APPROACH TO THE GROUND

A good example of this deception involves the nature of initial contact between the shoe and the ground. It is sometimes assumed that the foot approaches the ground rather as a helicopter approaches its landing pad, but that is far from the case as Fig. 2-1 indicates. Measurements taken by means of high-speed cinematography have shown that at the instant of foot strike* during running at 6.5 minutes per mile, the shoe may have a forward horizontal velocity component of 0.7 m/sec, or about 17% of the runner's average forward velocity. This velocity component can be combined vectorially with the vertical component of 0.75 m/sec to give a velocity of approach of approximately 1.1 m/sec. The values shown in Fig. 2-1 are average ones, and there is considerable variation between subjects. However, almost all subjects at their normal stride lengths are moving forward relative to the ground at foot strike.

---

*The term "foot strike" is used here in preference to the conventional term "heel strike" because the heel is not always the first part of the foot to make ground contact.

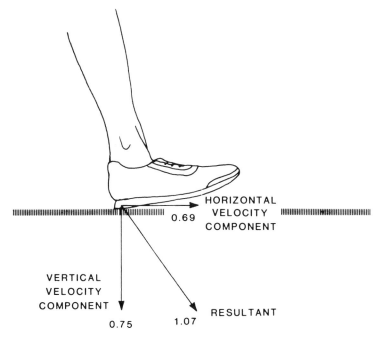

Fig. 2-1. Mean velocity components of heel immediately before foot strike in group of 10 subjects running at 6.5 minutes per mile (4.1 m/sec). Horizontal component of foot is almost as great as vertical (downward) component. Units are meters per second.

The forward motion at foot strike is evidenced by its effect on a runner's shoes. Some physicians absolutely forbid their patients to bring their old shoes to an office visit, and I think this is a mistake. Although I can understand the fear of having to listen to 10 minutes of history for each of 10 pairs of shoes, valuable information can be gained from well-worn shoes. Outsole wear does not occur because of high forces or pressures, and it is therefore wrong to identify a worn area on the shoe as the region of peak force. Abrasion occurs when there is relative movement between the shoe and the ground, and this is what happens at the instant of foot strike. The physician who looks at a variety of worn shoes will notice that there is invariably outsole wear somewhere along the lateral border of the shoe. In many cases this takes the form of a diagonal slice off the rear outside edge of the sole, indicating that this is the region where first ground contact is made. It is extremely rare to find wear on the posterior border of the running shoe, although this is common in shoes used for walking. Some runners have more well-defined lateral wear nearer the ball of the foot, indicating a distinctly different pattern of foot strike that I will discuss later in the chapter. Although these wear regions along the lateral border can give an indication of the most frequent site of initial contact, the terrain (particularly hill running), and the speed, they also tend to modify the foot strike in ways that have not been adequately studied.

MOVEMENTS AT FOOT STRIKE

Once initial contact with the ground has been made, external forces from the ground act on the body. I will consider the nature of these forces in a later section, but first I will describe the effects of these forces on joint motion.

Since the eye is an inadequate tool to measure rapid body motions, it is necessary to contrive some sort of measurement situation. This is generally done using high-speed cinematography of a subject running on a treadmill or over ground. The controversy over whether the two types of running are similar or different is largely irrelevant for the study of pathological gaits. Most scientists who have studied the problem have found subtle differences that are important in the study of the finer points of locomotor mechanics. However, it is unlikely that the foot strike is grossly different in treadmill running, and the convenience of being able to film many foot strikes outweighs minor differences.

Most attention has been directed to the motion of the rearfoot because it is the least mobile part of the foot and the easiest part to measure and also because it reflects the movement of the subtalar joint, which has been implicated in many running injuries, particularly knee injuries. Fig. 2-2 shows a typical situation for

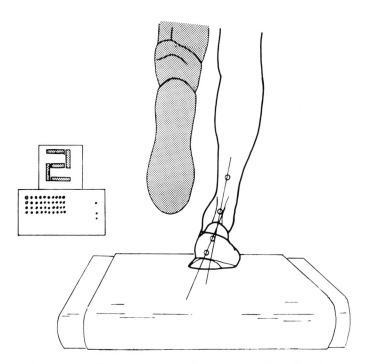

Fig. 2-2. Typical experimental situation for rearfoot motion analysis during running. Subject runs on treadmill, and markers are placed on posterior aspect of leg and shoe. Timing lights provide accurate time reference. Film will be subsequently digitized so that rearfoot angle plots like those shown in Fig. 2-3 can be obtained. This subject is in midsupport with everted foot, similar to subject 2 in Fig. 2-3.

measurement of rearfoot motion. Without three-dimensional cinematography, the measurements made are the projection of the markers placed on the shoe and leg in a frontal plane, and therefore the foot movements should be referred to as inversion and eversion.

　　Film must be taken at a rapid rate to measure the rapid movements that occur following foot strike. Frame rates of 200 to 400 frames per second are typically used. Once the film is taken, the markers on the body are converted to X-Y coordinates in an object-space reference frame by the process of frame-by-frame digitizing. A time reference is also taken from each frame of film so that precise temporal relationships can be determined. After the movement has been characterized in numerical form, angles can be calculated and plotted as shown in Fig. 2-3. It can be seen from the "normal" curve in Fig. 2-3 that the foot strike occurs with the

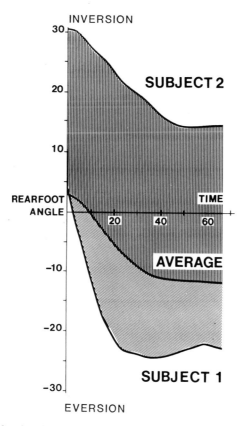

Fig. 2-3. Rearfoot angle plot showing average pattern of 10 subjects running at 6.5 minutes per mile. Foot starts in slight inversion at foot strike (time 0) and moves through range of motion of approximately 16 degrees in first 40 msec of contact phase. Subject 1 has excessive rearfoot motion. Subject 2 has normal range, but it occurs entirely in inversion region of curve.

ankle inverted to an average of 4 degrees. The tibialis anterior muscle is active during the swing to produce dorsiflexion of the foot, and it is also an inverter. As the graph shows, events occur rapidly as the foot strikes the ground. Eversion begins immediately, and within about 0.04 second (40 msec) an end point of eversion of approximately 12 degrees has been reached. Therefore the average foot has gone through a total range of motion of 16 degrees in only 0.04 second. This is the phase of subtalar joint pronation occurring in almost all normal runners immediately after foot strike. This pronation (combination of dorsiflexion and eversion) is an essential part of adapting to a plantigrade position, and it should certainly not be considered pathological.

Although the movement into eversion occurs rapidly, there is a "dwell" at the end point of the motion. This suggests that although high-speed data acquisition is necessary to map out the whole motion, less sophisticated equipment may be satisfactory to measure simply the end point. This offers the possibility that videotape equipment (with its conventional sampling rate of 30 complete scans per second) could be satisfactory for measurement of rearfoot motion in a clinical environment. Many physicians with a large number of runners in their practice have begun to include a treadmill and videotape recorder in their equipment.

What does an abnormal foot strike look like on these rearfoot angle plots? In Fig. 2-3 curves are presented for two individuals at opposite ends of the spectrum. Subject 1 has an excessive amount of rearfoot motion when compared to the mean curve, and subject 2 has a pattern that appears to be entirely in the inversion part of the graph. When the data were collected for subject 1, he was wearing an old pair of shoes with a badly battered heel counter and a midsole that had become compressed through wear. These features encouraged the subject's natural tendency to eversion, producing the excessive eversion seen in the curve. The curve shows that he continued to move into eversion over 10 degrees past the normal value and an astonishing 20 degrees beyond the neutral position. This runner was just beginning to experience lateral knee pain, which disappeared when he switched to a different pair of shoes. Subject 2 had very rigid feet, and his whole contact with the ground seemed to be on the outside border of the shoe. He was not, however, experiencing any pain. It is remarkable how frequently exaggerated patterns of rearfoot motion can be observed in pain-free runners. As suggested previously, these rearfoot angle curves depend to some degree on the shoe (and probably on the speed). Individuals with apparently excessive patterns of rearfoot motion when measured in their running shoes sometimes exhibit neutral patterns when running barefoot. This could be due to the assumption of a different running style by the subject when running barefoot, or it may be that measurements of the shoe are not a good indication of foot motion. A further possibility is that the beneficial cushioning properties of certain shoes have the detrimental feature of amplifying rearfoot motions that are small when the runner is barefoot. The property of limiting the change in rearfoot angle during ground contact is a major feature of the "rearfoot control" property of the shoe.

A look at the runner's shoes can be helpful in obtaining information concerning rearfoot motion in the absence of measuring equipment. The "table test" is a must for an examination of old shoes. The shoes are placed on a level table, and the heel region is viewed from behind. A valgus or varus alignment of the shoes suggests a corresponding misalignment of the rearfoot during support.

MOVEMENTS AT MIDSUPPORT

Once the steep part of the rearfoot angle curves in Fig. 2-3 has ended (a maximum of 0.05 second after foot strike), a large part of the sole of the shoe has come in contact with the ground and cinematography or videotape must be abandoned in the quest for information about shoe-ground interaction. These techniques no longer give much useful information because very little movement is occurring at this time.

It is, however, a mistake to regard the foot placement during midsupport as a static phenomenon. Wear under the forefoot region occurs because the support foot moves during weight-bearing. Some individuals have an exaggerated abductory twist of the foot in midsupport as the whole limb externally rotates. If this motion were to be totally resisted by, for example, long spikes on the outsole of the shoe, it is likely that the limb would undergo trauma or that the entire running style would have to be modified. The wear patterns that can be observed underneath the ball of the foot are an indication of the amount of motion that occurs during midsupport. In most runners, however, this twisting of the support foot is fairly small and difficult to observe.

The most frequently used method of learning what is happening underneath the foot in midsupport is force platform measurement. The force platform is rather like a complex bathroom scale, and the similarities between the two devices are useful in explaining how the force platform works. Both are based on the familiar Newton's third law of motion, which says that action and reaction are equal. When the weight and inertial force of the body act downward on the measuring device, an equal and opposite force known as the ground reaction force (GRF) acts upward on the body. The bathroom scale can measure only the vertical component of the GRF. Of course no locomotor movements can occur without components in the line of progression. The typical force platform is able to measure these components, sometimes called shear force components because they are parallel to the ground. The most important shear component is the anteroposterior one, which allows the runner to slow the body down during weight acceptance and accelerate it again during propulsion. Although the forces are measured at the feet, they should be thought of as acting on the center of mass of the body, since apart from air resistance and gravity they are the only external forces acting on the body.

We know from experience that on a bathroom scale it is possible to send the needle both above and below the body weight value by movements of body segments. A familiar example of reducing the GRF occurs in skiing as the skier unweights to make a parallel turn. The most obvious way to increase the GRF would be to jump down from a height. The value of the GRF changes in these examples because of Newton's second law. Sometimes expressed as $F = ma$, this law tells us that a force F must be acting on a body mass m that is accelerating by a units. The most important aspect of this law is the concept of "inertial forces," which explains why forces larger than body weight exist underneath the feet of a runner.

If the runner is in contact with the ground, a force of 1 times the body weight already exists because of the reaction of the ground to the pull of gravity on the body. But if the body is accelerating upward, there must be an additional force equal to ma acting in the same direction as the existing GRF. It is useful at this point to define upward acceleration. As the body weight is accepted by the supporting limb, the center of mass of the body is still traveling downward. Let us assume (based on measurements similar to those described earlier) that the center of mass has a downward (negative by convention) velocity of -1 m/sec. Moments later, as a result of the restraining action of the extensor musculature, it has a lesser velocity of, for example, -0.75 m/sec, still in a downward direction. The acceleration over this time interval(Δt) is

$$\frac{-0.75 - (-1.0)}{\Delta t} \text{ or } \frac{+0.25 \text{ units}}{\Delta t}$$

Since the sign is positive, the acceleration according to our convention is upward.

Later in the support phase the downward motion of the center mass has been halted completely (velocity 0), and in the next time interval (Δt) the center of mass is given a velocity of $+0.2$ m/sec upward (positive sign). The acceleration in the interval Δt was

$$\frac{0.2 - 0}{\Delta t} \text{ or } \frac{+0.2 \text{ units}}{\Delta t}$$

Again the sign is positive, indicating that an upward force must exist to sustain the upward acceleration.

By this fairly simple reasoning we have shown that the vertical component of the GRF is greater than the body weight for the majority of the contact phase. It should come as no surprise to see that this is indeed the case in Fig. 2-4. Let us follow in detail the events of this curve, which presents the average from 12 subjects running at 6.5 minutes per mile.

The curve is noticeably biphasic with an early peak of approximately twice body weight at about 20 msec (0.02 second) after foot strike and then a second peak approaching three times body weight at 80 msec. The entire contact with the ground lasts for only about 0.25 second. The two peaks have different rise times, the first very rapid and the second more gradual. The first peak is clearly associated with the impact of the foot strike, and as Fig. 2-3 indicates, pronation is still occurring as the impact peak subsides. It is somewhat surprising that this impact peak is actually smaller in magnitude than the second peak, which is associated with propulsion. The obvious suspicion cast on the force platform is unfounded because this

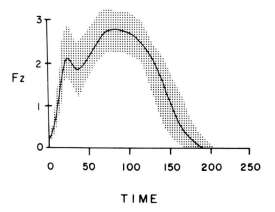

TIME

Fig. 2-4. Average vertical component of ground reaction force in 12 subjects running at 6.5 minutes per mile. Shaded area represents range of all subjects. Units of force (F_Z) are body weight, and time units are milliseconds (1/1000 second). Force rises to almost three times body weight and entire contact period lasts about 1/5 second.

REARFOOT

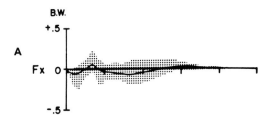

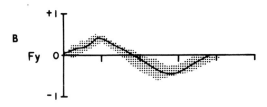

Fig. 2-5. Shear components of ground reaction force. **A,** Mediolateral. **B,** Anteroposterior. Note variability of mediolateral component and similarity in anteroposterior component in all subjects. Units are the same as those in Fig. 2-4, and data are from same subjects running at same speed. *B.W.,* body weight.

device is capable of responding to much more rapid change without significant attenuation.

Let us consider the findings of this simple experiment with the force platform in words rather than graphs. The static analogy to the dynamic findings just discussed would be for a 150-pound person to stand on the ball of one foot carrying an additional load of 300 pounds on his back. It is astounding that an activity as apparently innocuous as slow running results in such large forces between the shoe and the ground. These forces repeated over and over again produce the microtrauma that brings runners into orthopaedists' offices.

Fig. 2-5 shows typical patterns for the two shear components in the same group of runners running at the same speed as in Fig. 2-4. The shaded area indicates the variability in the sample.

The anteroposterior shear force has a fairly predictable shape. It builds up to a peak of approximately one-half body weight in a direction that tends to slow the runner down during the first part of the support phase. Then a smoothly rising force in the direction of progression indicates the steady push-off to regain the momentum lost during the braking phase. This second peak is of about the same magnitude as the first peak but of course is in the opposite direction. All subjects in the sample show approximately the same trends, and there is little difference in the peak values in terms of the subjects' body weights.

The mediolateral shear forces also shown in Fig. 2-5 present a very different situation. The striking feature of these curves is their variability. Further analysis of these data indicates that some subjects have a net impulse from the entire contact phase that is directed laterally, whereas other subjects have a net medially directed impulse. Thus it seems that it is in the mediolateral shear force direction that runners express their individuality. This is hardly surprising, considering the variety of foot placements with respect to the midline that exist in runners and the variety of anatomical characteristics that affect alignment. The relationships of these structural and style factors to the GRF recordings are not well understood and present a fruitful area for further research.

CENTER OF PRESSURE PATTERNS

In addition to measuring the magnitude and direction of the GRF, the force platform can provide information concerning the distribution of forces underneath the shoe. The quantity measured is called the center of pressure (COP), and this pressure point is a kind of average point of application of the applied force. Since forces are distributed over the sole of the shoe, the concept of a force applied at a point is potentially misleading. Nevertheless, it can give some insight until more elaborate techniques of measurement have been perfected.

The mean COP pattern for the entire contact phase of the group of runners whose data were presented previously is shown in Fig. 2-6. To understand this presentation, readers should imagine that they are looking down on their own right foot during the support phase of running. The shoe outline represents the mean

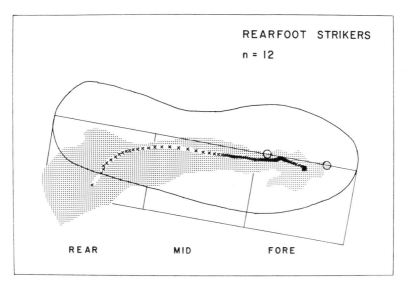

REARFOOT STRIKERS

n = 12

REAR   MID   FORE

Fig. 2-6. Center of pressure path for right foot in same group of runners as in Figs. 2-4 and 2-5. Crosses represent mean pattern (at 2-msec intervals), and shaded area is range from all subjects. See text for further details. (Reprinted with permission from J. Biomech., vol. 13, Cavanagh, P.R., and Lafortune, M.A., Ground reaction forces in distance running, Copyright 1980, Pergamon Press, Ltd.)

location of the foot during support (ignoring movements such as the abductory twist mentioned earlier). Each cross on the shoe outline represents the location of the COP in relation to the shoe at 2-msec intervals throughout the contact phase. The shaded area around the crosses indicates the range of locations measured from the 12 individuals studied. Because the measurements were equally spaced in time, some indication of the rate of progression of the COP across the shoe can be obtained from the illustration. Where the crosses are well separated, rapid transference of force was taking place. Where the crosses are bunched and indistinguishable from each other (as in the forefoot region), the situation was more stable and not much change in the distribution of pressure occurred.

Some of the factors that were previously discussed concerning shoe-ground interaction become clearer as we examine the COP plot. The display begins outside the shoe outline, showing clearly the scuffing that we hypothesized to occur at foot strike. Above-threshold values for force were already being recorded as the shoe scuffed across the ground to its final placement position. The typical outsole wear patterns mentioned previously are also consistent with the data in Fig. 2-6. The "trail" left by the shoe before placement is directed anteriorly and medially, suggesting some medial movement of the foot before foot strike in addition to the forward motion. Mediolateral movements of the foot have been inadequately studied to date.

From the range of points of inital contact it is clear that all of these subjects

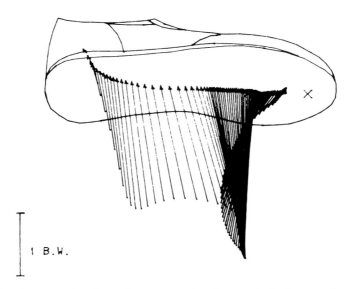

1 B.W.

Fig. 2-7. Resultant reaction forces (anteroposterior plus vertical) shown acting at center of pressure. See text for further details. *B.W.*, body weight. (Reprinted with permission from J. Biomech., vol. 13, Cavanagh, P.R., and Lafortune, M.A., Ground reaction forces in distance running, Copyright 1980, Pergamon Press, Ltd.)

could be classified as rearfoot strikers on the basis of the division of the shoe into rearfoot, midfoot, and forefoot sectors. The absence of initial contact on the posterior heel border mentioned earlier is clearly shown in Fig. 2-6.

Shortly after initial contact, the COP rapidly migrates medially and anteriorly until after about 50 msec it is at approximately 50% of shoe length from the heel. From this point until toe-off there is virtually no mediolateral migration in the COP path. There is also a distinct slowing of the rate of change of the COP as shown by the grouping of points, which become indistinguishable from each other. This dark region represents over two thirds of the contact phase, emphasizing the role that the forepart of the foot and shoe plays in running.

Since Figs. 2-4 and 2-6 represent data collected simultaneously for the same individuals, by matching the two data sets it is possible to show the force vectors associated with their respective COP patterns (Fig. 2-7). The previously mentioned limitations of the COP must be kept in mind when interpreting this correlation. It immediately becomes apparent in Fig. 2-7 that the largest peak in the vertical GRF appears at a time when the COP is under the forepart of the shoe. Because the vector underneath the shoe is a resultant of the vertical and anteroposterior components, the braking phase can be identified as the time when the force vectors are pointing backward and the propulsive phase as the time when they point forward. This further highlights the importance of forepart of the shoe, not only in protection of the foot but also in propulsion. Fig. 2-7 unifies much of the information concerning shoe-ground interaction presented so far.

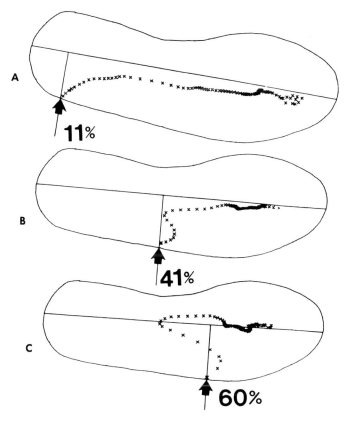

Fig. 2-8. Center of pressure patterns from three subjects all running at same speed. Note dramatic differences between subjects despite matched running speeds.

Other center of pressure patterns

The patterns of both force and COP discussed so far have been limited to the right feet of runners who were characterized as rearfoot strikers. The reader should not infer that these patterns are the only normal ones or that the left feet of these individuals would yield identical patterns. Fig. 2-8 shows three COP patterns collected from the right feet of runners moving between 6 and 6.5 minutes per mile. The graphs have been classified according to the point at which first contact between foot and shoe was made. This value is expressed as a percentage of shoe length to give a "strike index" for the individual. The strike index varies from 11% to 60% in these three individuals. These are not contrived patterns but real differences between the running styles of individuals. The different patterns imply a distinctly different loading history and also different requirements in footwear for individuals with rearfoot, midfoot, and forefoot strikes at the same speed of running. Speed also alters the COP pattern, but the effect of speed has been overemphasized in the past. Previously the patterns shown in Fig. 2-8, *A, B,* and *C,* might have been attributed to jogging, middle-distance running, and short-distance running speeds, respectively. It now appears that individual differences are at least as important as speed. Force-time curves such as those in Figs. 2-4 and 2-5 also exhibit special features depending on the foot strike. For example, midfoot strikers show less prominent initial peaks in the vertical GRF curves but have a biphasic anteroposterior component during braking.

Concerning symmetry, the pair of COP patterns in Fig. 2-9 is of interest. They represent the left and right feet of marathon runner Bill Rodgers running at his race pace of 5 minutes per mile. Rodgers is clearly a toe runner; cinematographic data

BILL RODGERS 5 MIN LT.

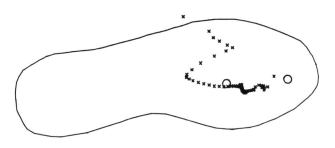

BILL RODGERS 5 MIN RT.

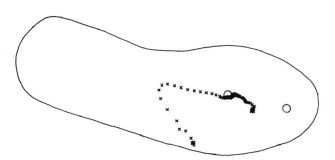

Fig. 2-9. Center of pressure patterns from left and right feet of marathon runner Bill Rodgers during running at 5 minute per mile pace. Note bilateral asymmetry.

confirm that on level ground his left heel does not touch the ground. But the patterns of pressure distribution under the left and right feet are very different, and this may be related to the fact that Rodgers' left leg is approximately 1 cm shorter than his right. Minor asymmetries in the COP patterns are fairly common in our experimental subjects, and their significance should be studied further.

MAPPING THE ENTIRE SHOE-GROUND INTERFACE

As suggested previously, the COP pattern provides an interesting but not completely adequate description of the shoe-ground interface. The problem is the res-

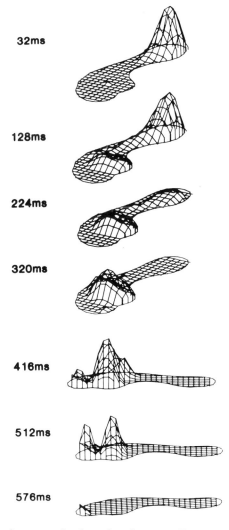

Fig. 2-10. Pressure distribution under bare foot during walking. See text for further details. (From Clarke, T.E.: The pressure distribution under the foot during barefoot walking, Ph.D. thesis, The Pennsylvania State University, University Park, 1980.)

olution and identification of peak pressures with anatomical structures of the foot. There has been sporadic interest in the problem of mapping the entire shoe-ground interface over the last 50 years, but only recently has the equipment been available to perform a satisfactory analysis. Unfortunately, none of the methods has yet been applied to running, although studies in the Biomechanics Laboratory at Pennsylvania State University are close to achieving this goal. An example of what might be expected is shown in Fig. 2-10 from the work of Clarke.[3] This figure represents a sequence of pressure distribution plots collected during slow, barefoot walking. The height of the display above the ground plane is proportional to the pressure at that location. With such a display, the association between observation and anatomical structures is considerably enhanced.

CONCLUSION

The aim of this chapter has been to show that the techniques of biomechanical measurement can produce considerable information about the interface of the shoe with the ground during running. So far mostly symptom-free subjects have been examined, but the results are encouraging enough to consider proceeding with the next step: applying the techniques described to a large number of patients who have been subjected to a thorough clinical analysis and grouped according to well-defined clinical entities. Running injuries are exceedingly subtle phenomena, and the results of experiments on runners are unlikely to provide an immediate guide to diagnosis or prophylaxis. However, biomechanical measurement must become an integral part of orthopaedic medicine, since the orthopaedist, more than most other physicians, works heavily under the influence of Newton's laws.

REFERENCES

1. Cavanagh, P.R.: The running shoe book, Mountain View, Calif., 1980, Anderson World.
2. Cavanagh, P.R., and Lafortune, M.A.: Ground reaction forces in distance running, J. Biomech. **13:**397, 1980.
3. Clarke, T.E.: The pressure distribution under the foot during barefoot walking, Ph.D. thesis, The Pennsylvania State University, University Park, 1980.

3. Basic cardiovascular physiology — development of a personal conditioning program

Kenneth H. Cooper

LIFE-STYLE CHANGE IN THE 1970s

A significant change occurred in American life-styles during the 1970s. A 1961 Gallup poll estimated that less than 24% of the adult population exercised regularly and fewer than 100,000 people were jogging. The statistics were about the same in 1968, that is, 24% were exercising regularly and slightly more than 100,000 were jogging. During the next decade, however, something happened to increase the number of exercisers so that in 1977 a Gallup poll estimated that 47% of the American population were participating in some type of daily physical exercise. An estimated 27 to 30 million Americans were jogging one to three times a week in 1977.

The 1977 Gallup poll revealed that the upper socioeconomic groups were more likely to exercise. Individuals under 30 years of age were more likely to exercise than those over 30, and men exercised more regularly than women. Demographically, joggers tended to be single, young, college educated, and in the upper-middle income brackets and to live in the Northeast and Far West regions of the United States. The exercise boom and subsequent life-style change have occurred not only in the United States but in several foreign countries. As evidence of this, the aerobics books have been translated into 20 foreign languages and nearly 12 million copies have been sold.

HEALTH BENEFITS OF EXERCISE

It is imperative that changes in health patterns be examined for possible associations between health benefits and exercise. The expected increased incidence in heart attacks has not occurred. In fact, there was a 23% decrease in deaths from heart attacks from 1968 to 1978. If the incidence of cardiovascular deaths projected in 1968 had occurred, there would have been an estimated 164,000 additional deaths in 1978. In addition to the decrease in mortality from heart attacks, other benefits are noteworthy. For example, from 1968 to 1978 there was a 36% decrease in deaths from cerebrovascular accidents and a 48% decrease in deaths from hypertensive disease.

The decade of the 1970s is also associated with a significant increase in life span, but whether this is coincidental or related to the increased participation in exercise is unknown. The average American's longevity was increased 2.7 years to a total of 73.2 years—an increase of almost three times the usual 1-year increase of earlier decades. A major reason for this increase in life span, according to Surgeon General Julius B. Richmond, is the marked reduction in deaths from cardiovascular disease, the nation's leading killer. At this time we can only assume that a change in exercise habits has contributed to the aforementioned health gains in America, but it is apparent that the practice of preventive medicine is beginning to have a significant impact on our society.

HEALTH CARE COSTS

It is encouraging to realize that the cost of health care can be reduced by a greater interest in preventive medicine. In 1950 the estimated annual cost of health care in the United States was $12 billion. In 1970 the health care cost was $70 billion, and in 1978 it was $192 billion. At the Healthy America Conference in Washington, D.C., in June 1980, Senator Robert Dole projected the cost of health care at more than $240 billion in the 1980s. Senator Dole further explained that 3% of the $240 billion will be spent on prevention of disease and 97% on treatment.

An issue frequently debated in the United States is whether national health insurance will improve the health of the American people. It is important to note that the improvements in health during the last decade have been accomplished without a national health insurance program. According to Richard E. Palmer, past president of the American Medical Association,

> The medical system affects only 10% of the usual factors that determine a patient's state of health—the remaining 90% are determined by factors over which doctors have little or no control. Physicians maintain that more sensible personal health decisions on smoking, drinking, exercise, and proper diet offer better hope for a healthier American than a sweeping restructuring of the medical system.[10]

Another problem, as stated by the American Health Foundation, is that "ours is a legacy of a medical system which provides too much care too late. Clearly, a new approach is needed and that approach must concentrate on the practice of preventive medicine."[2]

Why do people neglect preventive medicine and fail to take advantage of its obvious health benefits and savings in health care costs? According to a feature story by Ashley Montague in the *New York Times,*

> The health of the people should surely be our number one priority; yet, we show little interest in this. Preventive medicine after years of struggle to stay alive remains the Cinderella of the medical specialties. . . . Too many of us will not see a doctor when we are well for fear that something may be discovered that is wrong with us. Most people regard health

as something one goes to the doctor to be restored when one is sick. Hence, health becomes a function of disease and one sees a doctor only when one is sick. Furthermore, doctors on the whole are uninterested in health since their training is focused virtually entirely on disease and there is very little profit in health.[9]

CORONARY RISK FACTORS

The leading cause of death in Americans is coronary artery disease. There are indications, however, that with maintenance of ideal body weight, proper diet, abstinence from tobacco, and proper exercise the death rate from cardiovascular disease can be reduced.

It is exciting to look at the association between coronary risk factors and physical fitness levels. This observation suggests the role that exercise can play in preventive medicine.

The Cooper Clinic in Dallas evaluated nearly 3000 men during the years 1971 to 1974. Of these patients, 8% were less than 30 years of age; 30% were between 30 and 39; 37% were between 40 and 49; 20% were between 50 and 59; and 5% were more than 60. In general the patients were self-referrals. Of this patient population 40% lived outside the Dallas/Fort Worth area and 0.9% lived outside the United States; 70.6% were college graduates. Before testing, each subject completed an extensive medical history questionnaire that included general information, occupation, purpose for coming to the clinic, present and past medical history, family history, smoking, and exercise habits.

The subjects reported to the Cooper Clinic for morning testing after a 12-hour fast. They were asked not to smoke before coming to the laboratory. All tests were conducted in air-conditioned rooms with an ambient temperature of $22° ± 3°$ C. A 15-ml blood sample drawn from the antecubital vein after 15 to 20 minutes of rest was analyzed for serum cholesterol, triglyceride, glucose, and uric acid levels. Cholesterol, glucose, and uric acid values were determined with an automated analysis system. Serum triglyceride values were determined with a single-channel automated system according to the method described by Kessler and Lederer.[6] The high-density lipoprotein (HDL) cholesterol value was determined by using an ABA-100 analyzer after very low–density lipoprotein (VLDL) and low-density lipoprotein (LDL) cholesterol were precipitated with sodium phosphotungstate in the presence of magnesium chloride. The LDL-plus-VLDL cholesterol value was calculated by subtracting the HDL cholesterol value from the total cholesterol value. Standard samples were used for daily checks on the blood analyzers, and quality control checks were made monthly.

With subjects in a standing position, the forced vital capacity was determined using a spirometer. The residual volume measure, used in the equation for estimating body density, was estimated from both height and age as outlined by Goldman and Becklace.[5] The methods for spirometry calculations were those recommended by Korey, Callahan, and Boren.[7]

With the subjects in the nude, a standard physician's scale was used to measure body weight to the nearest 0.10 kg and height to the nearest 0.16 cm. To ensure the accuracy of the body density measurement, which was determined by the underwater displacement technique described by Allen,[1] each subject underwent multiple trials. Then, using the equation of Brozek and co-workers,[4] the percentage of body fat was calculated from the body density measurement.

After a rest period of approximately 10 minutes, a standard 12-lead supine electrocardiogram was recorded. Abnormal resting electrocardiograms were tabulated, and patients with severe problems that might be enhanced by stress testing were excluded from the study. Resting heart rates were obtained from a 6-second recording of a standard V_5 electrocardiographic lead while the patient was at rest in the supine position. Systolic and diastolic blood pressure readings were taken with the patient in the sitting position. All blood pressure tests were performed using a calibrated aneroid sphygmomanometer.

Cardiorespiratory endurance was determined from a maximum treadmill stress test according to a modified Balke and Ware protocol.[3] The grade of the treadmill was level for the first minute, elevated 2% at the end of the first minute, and subsequently increased 1% per minute until the twenty-fifth minute. The speed of the treadmill was held constant at 90 m/min (3.3 miles per hour) until the twenty-fifth minute. At that point the speed was increased 0.2 miles per hour each minute until the termination of the test. Each subject was instructed to continue the stress test for as long as possible. Volitional exhaustion, electrocardiographic abnormality, or a minimum of 85% of the age-adjusted predicted maximum heart rate were the end points for the maximum treadmill stress test. If the test was terminated before the desired maximum heart rate was reached because of severe chest pain, abnormally high or low blood pressure, ataxia, vertigo, or an abnormal electrocardiogram, the patient was eliminated from the study.

Age-adjusted performance time categories as listed in Table 3-1 determined the level of cardiorespiratory fitness. These standards are based on the relationship between treadmill time and maximum oxygen consumption and a standard distribution of subject performance.

Table 3-1. Cardiorespiratory fitness levels for men*

Fitness level	Treadmill stress test time (min:sec)				
	<30 yr	30-39 yr	40-49 yr	50-59 yr	60+ yr
Very poor	<12:00	<11:00	<10:00	<9:00	<8:00
Poor	12:00-14:59	11:00-13:59	10:00-12:59	9:00-11:59	8:00-10:59
Fair	15:00-17:59	14:00-16:59	13:00-15:59	12:00-14:59	11:00-13:59
Good	18:00-21:59	17:00-20:59	16:00-19:59	15:00-18:59	14:00-17:59
Excellent	>22:00	>21:00	>20:00	>19:00	>18:00

*Based on a modified Balke treadmill stress test protocol and levels of fitness developed at the Institute for Aerobics Research, 1974.

Tables 3-2 and 3-3 compare cardiorespiratory fitness with selected physiological and coronary risk factor measures. Only significant differences as related to the excellent level of fitness are included. No significant differences between the good and excellent levels of fitness were found in the intergroup comparisons except for serum triglyceride levels and percentage of body fat. Further analyses demonstrated a significant difference between the very poor and poor categories of fitness in blood glucose levels, systolic and diastolic blood pressure, and percentage of body fat. The good and fair levels of fitness differed significantly in serum cholesterol and triglyceride levels, uric acid concentration, systolic and diastolic blood pressure, and percentage of body fat. Interestingly, there was a significant relationship between forced vital capacity and level of cardiorespiratory fitness when these values were adjusted for age, height, weight, and percentage of body fat.

HDL cholesterol and LDL-plus-VLDL cholesterol values for two subgroups of men ranging in age from 40 to 49 years are presented in Tables 3-4 and 3-5, respectively. Compared to the data presented in Tables 3-2 and 3-3, the same relationships between levels of fitness and HDL cholesterol and LDL-plus-VLDL cholesterol are present. Highly significant differences ($p<.01$) were found between the excellent fitness level group and all other groups for these variables. Thus patients with excellent fitness have a lower coronary disease risk because of their higher HDL cholesterol levels and lower LDL-plus-VLDL cholesterol levels.

An inverse relationship between levels of cardiorespiratory fitness and variables

Table 3-2. Physical fitness levels versus selected physiological variables

Level of physical fitness	Age (yr) (N = 2924)	Height (cm) (N = 2622)	Weight (kg) (N = 2685)	Heart rate* (beats/min) (N = 2904)	Forced vital capacity (L) (N = 2502)
Very poor					
$\overline{X}$	48.2†	176.8	90.0†	69.7†	4.3†
n	351	316	323	349	300
Poor					
$\overline{X}$	44.0	178.1	86.3†	66.3†	4.6†
n	585	544	551	578	525
Fair					
$\overline{X}$	42.3	178.7	82.8†	64.0†	5.0†
n	876	801	817	871	770
Good					
$\overline{X}$	40.6	179.1	79.4‡	59.5†	5.1†
n	802	707	728	797	674
Excellent					
$\overline{X}$	40.7	178.9	76.2	51.6	5.3
n	310	254	266	306	233

*Resting, sitting values.
†$p<.01$ when compared to the excellent level of physical fitness.
‡$p<.05$ when compared to the excellent level of physical fitness.

Table 3-3. Physical fitness levels versus selected coronary risk factors

Level of physical fitness	Cholesterol (mg/100 ml) (N = 2514)	Triglycerides (ml/100 ml) (N = 2477)	Glucose (mg/100 ml) (N = 2468)	Uric acid (mg/100 ml) (N = 2472)	Blood pressure (mm Hg)*		Body fat (%) (N = 2266)
					Systolic (N = 2905)	Diastolic (N = 2905)	
Very poor							
$\overline{X}$	237.1†	182.1‡	112.8‡	6.9‡	132.6‡	86.6†	29.3‡
	(229.9†)§	(176.8‡)	(111.0‡)	(6.7†)	(127.6‡)	(83.4)	(26.1‡)
n	294	290	290	290	348	348	241
Poor							
$\overline{X}$	238.5‡	171.6‡	107.7‡	7.0‡	126.5†	83.8†	26.9‡
	(232.9‡)	(163.8‡)	(107.3‡)	(6.8‡)	(124.9)	(82.4)	(25.3‡)
n	530	523	522	523	580	580	477
Fair							
$\overline{X}$	228.8†	104.4‡	105.5†	6.8‡	124.6†	83.2†	24.0‡
	(226.9)	(138.7‡)	(105.6)	(6.7†)	(124.4)	(82.2)	(24.0‡)
n	767	759	755	758	871	871	711
Good							
$\overline{X}$	222.9	114.3‡	104.0	6.5	122.5	80.9	20.8‡
	(225.1)	(118.9‡)	(105.3)	(6.5)	(123.4)	(81.9)	(22.4‡)
n	670	665	663	663	797	797	620
Excellent							
$\overline{X}$	217.3	87.4	102.1	6.3	122.1	79.8	18.2
	(221.1)	(98.3)	(103.4)	(6.4)	(122.9)	(81.4)	(20.8)
n	253	240	238	238	309	309	217

*Resting, sitting values.
†$p < .05$ when compared to the excellent level of physical fitness.
‡$p < .01$ when compared to the excellent level of physical fitness.
§Scores in parentheses adjusted for age, body weight, and percentage of body fat.

Table 3-4. Fitness versus HDL cholesterol level in 732 men*

Fitness category†	n	Mean HDL cholesterol level (mg/100 ml)
Very poor	45	37.0‡
Poor	103	40.5‡
Fair	188	41.5‡
Good	222	44.5‡
Excellent	174	49.3

*First visit; average age 45 years.
†From age-adjusted, maximum performance treadmill stress test time, Balke protocol.
‡Significant when compared to excellent ($p < .01$).

Table 3-5. Fitness versus LDL-plus-VLDL cholesterol level in 709 men*

Fitness category†	n	Mean LDL-plus-VLDL cholesterol level (mg/100 ml)
Very poor	44	185.5‡
Poor	101	186.6‡
Fair	180	172.0‡
Good	215	171.8‡
Excellent	169	161.9

*First visit; average age 45 years.
†From age-adjusted, maximum performance treadmill stress test time, Balke protocol.
‡Significant when compared to excellent ($p<.01$).

Table 3-6. Risk factor changes and fitness improvement*

Cholesterol	− 11.0 mg/100 ml
Triglycerides	− 14.4 mg/100 ml
Glucose	− 8.3 mg/100 ml
Systolic blood pressure	− 2.1 mm Hg
Diastolic blood pressure	− 2.6 mm Hg
Body fat	− 0.2%
Treadmill time	+ 1.7 min

*After 30.3 months in 1499 men aged 30 to 59 years.

Table 3-7. Risk factor changes in top 10% and lowest 10% of fitness improvement groups (men 30 to 59 years of age)

Risk factor	Least improvement (150 patients)	Most improvement (150 patients)
Glucose (mg/dl)	− 7.0	− 10.6*
Triglycerides (mg/dl)	7.5	− 63.3†
Cholesterol (mg/dl)	2.3	− 22.9†
Systolic blood pressure (mm Hg)	1.3	− 4.6†
Diastolic blood pressure (mm Hg)	− 1.1	− 4.9†
Body fat (%)	3.4	− 2.8†

*$p<.05$.
†$p<.001$.

related to a higher coronary disease risk is presented in Tables 3-2 to 3-5. A criticism of this cross-sectional data might be that those in the excellent category of fitness already had lower coronary risk factors while those in the poor category of fitness had high risk factors. In an effort to answer this question, 1499 healthy men volunteered to participate in a longitudinal study to document changes in coronary risk factors with exercise. Using the previously mentioned methods, baseline blood values and levels of physical fitness were determined. These volunteers, who averaged 44.6 years of age, were carefully followed for 30.3 months. At the end of the study their treadmill performance time had increased an average of 1.7 minutes. Changes in their coronary risk factors are documented in Table 3-6.

No participants were excluded from this study, even though some of the participants admittedly did not exercise during the 30 months. A comparison of the top 10% with the lowest 10% revealed interesting findings (Table 3-7). A significant decrease was noted in the coronary risk factors in those who improved their physical fitness level the most. Body weight loss was also significantly related to risk factor changes, but subsequent analysis showed that fitness improvement remained significantly related to reduced risk even after body weight loss was statistically controlled by partial correlations.

STRESS TESTING, THE BEST PREDICTOR

A group of 126 patients, among the 20,000 patients visiting the Cooper Clinic during the last 10 years, had a major coronary event within a few months to 2 years after their fitness evaluation. The average age of these patients was 57 years. They were unique because nearly all of them thought they were healthy when they came to the clinic, and they desired to maintain good health. They died suddenly of what was diagnosed as a heart attack, had a heart attack and survived, or required coronary artery bypass surgery. By looking at the risk factors listed by the American Heart Association and trying to determine the best predictor of these major coronary problems, we discovered the following.

Of the 126 patients, 31 had a fasting blood sugar level greater than 110 mg/100 ml; 49 had triglyceride levels greater than 150 mg/100 ml; 44 were current cigarette smokers; 49 had a family member who had had a heart attack at less than 50 years of age; 80 were overweight (over 19% body fat as determined by underwater weighing or skin caliper measurements or both); 51 had blood pressures greater than 140/90 mm Hg at the time of their first evaluation; 65 had cholesterol levels greater than 250 mg/100 ml; 35 had an abnormal resting electrocardiogram*; and 76 had an abnormal stress electrocardiogram. In over 41,000 maximum performance treadmill stress tests at the Aerobics Center in Dallas, 11% of patients with a normal resting electrocardiogram had a grossly abnormal stress test, showing that some people with normal resting electrocardiograms have serious disease problems that would

---

*Resting electrocardiograms are poor predictors of impending major coronary problems.

not be diagnosed except by stress testing. Since the sensitivity and specificity of our tests are high, false-positive and false-negative results are unusual.

Yet, the best predictor of impending coronary heart disease and probably the best indicator of protection against coronary heart disease may be the treadmill test time. Of the 126 who later had coronary events, 101 could not meet a fitness threshold of 15 minutes using the standard Balke treadmill protocol, which is the first level believed to offer some protection against coronary heart disease. A period of 15 minutes using the Balke protocol is equivalent to running 2 miles in 20 minutes.

In a study reported by Margolis and co-workers[8] of Duke University Medical School, 1250 patients with chest pain came to their clinic for a diagnostic workup. As part of the diagnostic evaluation, these patients had both coronary arteriography and a treadmill stress test. The coronary arteriograms revealed that 744 patients in this group had one-, two-, or three-vessel obstructive coronary disease. After following these patients with checks made at 6-, 12-, 24-, and 36-month intervals, it was discovered that for those who could walk longer than 15 minutes using a Balke protocol (level IV Bruce protocol), the mortality was only 2% during the next 3 years, whereas for those who could not walk longer than 7 minutes using a Balke protocol (level I Bruce protocol), the mortality was greater than 41% during the next 2 years. Although all of these patients had obstructive coronary heart disease, the compensation in the former group was adequate and they did not need bypass surgery. For the others, bypass surgery may have been lifesaving; therefore the level of fitness may be not only an independent variable in coronary disease but one of the most important variables.

Treadmill stress testing is very valuable in diagnostic cardiology and is safe if performed properly and if patients are selected carefully and watched closely during the testing. Most stress testing, however, does not bring the subject to exhaustion and is inadequately monitored. Only maximum performance stress testing with multiple-lead monitoring is performed at the Cooper Clinic. With this system, all 12 of the standard electrocardiographic leads plus the three leads of the vectorcardiogram are monitored, which increases the sensitivity and specificity of stress testing. The treadmill technique used at the Cooper Clinic is a modified Balke protocol, which takes about twice as long as the Bruce protocol and gives the patient a longer warm-up period. For example, 15 minutes with the Bruce test is equivalent to 25 minutes with the Balke test.[11] Consequently, the Bruce protocol is more commonly used in stress testing laboratories.

The most important reason for stress testing is to determine whether the patient has signs of obstructive coronary artery disease. In over 41,000 maximum performance treadmill stress tests at the Cooper Clinic, only one patient required electrical defibrillation. This occurred in January 1975 when a 49-year-old man visited the clinic for a physical examination. At rest his electrocardiogram was normal, but as soon as stress testing began, a depression of the J point was noticed. At first there was no typical flattening or depression of the ST segment, but as he continued to exercise, classic flattening of the ST segments in multiple leads was noted. After 14 minutes the treadmill test was stopped; the patient's maximum heart rate had reached only 145 beats per minute. Unlike most laboratories conducting stress tests, the Cooper Clinic does not stop its testing abruptly. Patients are asked to walk slowly for an additional 3 minutes, since the majority of arrhythmias associated with exercise occur during recovery and not during the exercise itself. As much as 60% of a person's blood may be pooled below the waist at the conclusion of vigorous exercise. Because of inadequate cerebral circulation, fainting may occur if an individual stops abruptly and stands motionless.

When a patient reaches exhaustion, he grasps the bar* and the incline is gradually lowered with the speed reduced from 3.3 to 1.5 miles per hour for the 3-minute walking cool down period. The patient is then asked to lie down or sit down for the next 7 to 10 minutes while being monitored continuously. After the required 3 minutes, the patient who required defibrillation sat down and his heart rate dropped to 53 beats per minute. This type of bradycardia is seen in world-class athletes or in patients who have sick hearts. As a further indication of this man's sick heart, he began to have multiple ectopic beats. Then at 4 minutes and 45 seconds into recovery, he lapsed into unconsciousness as classic ventricular tachycardia and fibrillation occurred following a malignant premature ventricular contraction (PVC). (By definition, a malignant PVC occurs on the peak or the downslope of the T wave). He did not respond to mouth-to-mouth resuscitation or closed chest cardiac massage. Therefore he was given a single 400 watt/sec shock. This almost worked; however, ventricular tachycardia returned and a second shock was necessary. The patient's rhythm then returned to normal, although initially it was very slow. He was given intravenous medications including lidocaine and sodium bicarbonate, and his heart rate was stabilized at 120 beats per minute. He regained consciousness and was taken to a nearby hospital for observation. Further studies showed no signs of myocardial infarction, no enzyme changes, no electrocardiographic changes, and no indication of permanent damage—literally a heart "too good to die." Only coronary arteriography revealed the real problem, which was corrected by multiple-vessel bypass surgery.

SUMMARY

During the 1970s, considerable advances were made in the use of exercise in the practice of diagnostic and therapeutic medicine. It is encouraging that many attempts are now being made to quantify the role of exercise in preventive medicine. As stated by Carlton Chapman, past president of the American Heart Association, "The use of exercise in the prevention, diagnosis, and rehabilitation of patients with cardiovascular disease is in a state of transition from unfounded faddism to scientific legitimacy." At the Institute for Aerobics Research in Dallas, the results

---

*Patients are not allowed to hold on to the bar during exercise testing because this decreases the energy cost and thus invalidates the fitness measurement.

in studying 20,000 patients have provided data that are bridging the gap between faddism and scientific legitimacy and that strongly encourage exercise as an integral part of today's life-style.

REFERENCES

1. Allen, T.H.: Measurement of human body fat: a quantitative method suited for use by aviation medical officers, Aerospace Med. **43:**907, 1963.
2. American Health Foundation: Unpublished statement.
3. Balke, B., and Ware, R.: An experimental study of physical fitness of Air Force personnel, U.S. Armed Forces Med. J. **10:**675, 1959.
4. Brozek, J., and others: Densitometric analysis of body composition: revision of some quantitative assumptions, Ann. N.Y. Acad. Sci. **110:**113, 1963.
5. Goldman, H.I., and Becklace, M.R.: Respiratory function tests: normal values at medium altitudes and the prediction of normal results, Am. Rev. Tuberc. Resp. Dis. **79:**457, 1959.
6. Kessler, G., and Lederer, H.: Fluorometric measurement of triglycerides. In Skeggs, L.T., editor: Automation in analytical chemistry, Technicon Symposium, 1965, New York, 1966, Mediad, Inc.
7. Kory, R., Callahan, R., and Boren, H.: The Veteran's Administration–Army cooperative study of pulmonary function, Am. J. Med. **30:**243, 1961.
8. Margolis, J.R.: Presentation at the American Heart Association Meeting, Raleigh, N.C., 1976.
9. Montague, A.: Rehumanizing medicine, New York Times, December 1, 1975.
10. Palmer, R.E.: Newsweek, June 6, 1977.
11. Pollock, M.L., and others: A comparative analysis of four protocols for maximal treadmill stress testing, Am. Heart J. **92:**39, 1976.

4. Prescription for the beginner

William J. Bowerman

If a little is good, is more better and is the limit best? Certainly not, especially in the area of exercise!

Since the people of the United States and the world have taken to the streets, many have tried to increase their running mileage to 100 to 150 miles per week. I have two quick rebuttals to the 100 miles per week theories of training. First, I have never coached a really successful runner whose regular training included more than 70 miles per week, and this includes 17 sub-4-minute milers, 5 champion 3-milers, and 2 world-class marathoners. Second, among those who insisted on training with longer distances there were no champions and a high proportion of physical breakdowns. I coached one 4:00.2-minute miler who could never run more than 25 miles per week without suffering some minor or major physical disability but who maintained his maximum health and fitness on the 25 miles per week program.

Training *principles* are the same for people of all ages and expectations. Training *practices* (such as fartlek, intervals, and steady-state running) are flexible, their amounts and frequency varying according to the ability and goals of each individual.

TRAINING SCHEDULE

My method of devising a training schedule (specific assignments for workouts) is not very different from a physician's method of arriving at a prescription for a patient. The first step is diagnosis, becoming acquainted with the patient's or athlete's abilities and disabilities. The second step is an assessment of what improvement can reasonably be expected and what specific recommendations are needed. The final step is a period of trial and observation to adjust the "dosage" or training schedule to optimum levels for the safest and most rapid improvement of condition.

Beginners, particularly unfit middle-aged adults of sedentary habits or individuals seeking rehabilitation after illness or injury, should have a thorough examination by a qualified physician to find out if there are any special limitations on activity.

If there are no outwardly imposed limitations, a test is given to determine the individual's level of ability. The results of the test establish a time for covering certain distances in the training routines for the next few weeks. At the end of that time another test indicates readiness for increasing distance and decreasing time (adding more stress) in subsequent workouts.

When Dr. Waldo Harris, a Eugene, Oregon, cardiologist and internist, and I performed our original experiments with mixed groups of adult joggers, we began with 2 weeks of easy conditioning before the first test efforts. This period allowed the joggers to recover from minor stiffness and develop self-confidence and an understanding of what they should expect to accomplish. This also allowed us to observe the joggers and divide them into three ability classifications to prevent undue competitiveness or discouragement.

After the initial 2 weeks' conditioning, our joggers began exactly as the runners I train do at the beginning of each new season, with a test to see if they could cover 880 yards (½ mile) without strain. When working with runners, I suggest that they go through the test at three-fourths maximum effort. With beginners, who would probably be unable to judge what this means, I explain,

Make two complete circuits of the track, which will be ½ mile, at a pace well within your tolerance. Whenever you feel your pace is too fast, slow down or even walk. When comfortable, resume a quicker pace. You will be timed for the half mile. One eighth of your total time, or the average time you took to cover 110 yards, will be your training pace, the basis for your assignments for the next 2 weeks.

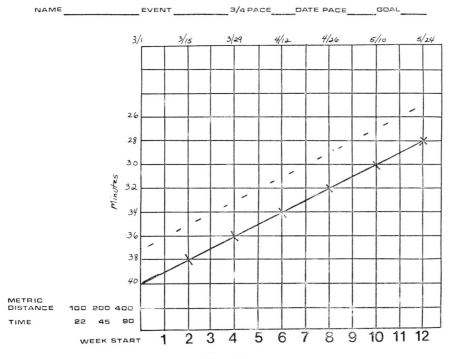

Fig. 4-1

When I am working with only one person, I do the timing myself. When working with a group, as we did in the jogging study, I ask the group to count off by two's to establish partners. When the "one's" are running, the "two's" listen to the official timer who calls out the times as joggers finish their two laps. Each "two" is responsible for recording and reporting his partner's finish time. Likewise, when the "two's" run, their partners record and report their times.

After a runner or jogger has ascertained his training or *date pace*, it is entered on a graph as the first X in the lower left corner (Fig. 4-1). In the upper right corner another X is placed to indicate the *goal pace*, which represents the time in which an individual (or his coach, trainer, physician, or adviser) believes he will be able to run the same distance 3 months later. The numbers running upward on the left margin of the graph start with the date pace and progress to the goal pace at the top of the column. The numbers across the top of the graph are the dates at 2-week intervals for the following 3 months. On each of these dates another test effort will be run. A diagonal line drawn from the date pace at the bottom left to the last date at the upper right indicates the jogger's expected rate of progress. Lines drawn across the graph from the pace numbers intersect the progress line and the perpendicular lines from the various dates to show the pace at which the jogger should expect to cover 110 yards of another 880-yard run on each testing date.

This kind of chart provides the runner and his adviser with a simple way to assess progress and to adjust the training schedule as necessary.

SETS OF EXERCISE

The most important question is: How does the runner or jogger get from the first X on the chart to the final X? The answer: By practicing a regularly repeated but varied set of exercises, which should be written out in advance in accordance with a master plan on a schedule.

On this schedule every other day should consist of light exercise, not more than 20 minutes of easy jogging, swimming, weight-lifting, walking, bicycling, or whatever is pleasurable. Serious or "hard" workouts take place on the alternate days. Even these hard workouts, however, should adhere to the maxim "Train, don't strain."[2]

Serious workouts generally consist of intervals, fartlek, steady-state running, or a combination of these with appropriate variations.

Interval work is running or jogging comparatively short distances, which are repeated a specified number of times with appropriate rest intervals of walking or easy jogging. A beginner should probably start with intervals of about 55 yards, repeated not more than four times at his date pace with whatever rest he needs in between to recover normal breathing and pulse rate. Over a 3-month period most beginners work up to intervals of 220 yards or even 440 yards (once around a quarter-mile track), repeated as many as six times. Those who are young, comparatively fit, and well acquainted with their own tolerance for exercise and stress will probably be able to take on more than this moderate schedule.

Fartlek is a Scandinavian word meaning speed play. Fartlek is assigned by the length of time it is to be practiced rather than by a distance to be covered. During 20 to 45 minutes of fartlek a runner may include any or all elements of a race, increasing or decreasing his speed whenever he wishes and adding, if he likes, special exercises such as jumping, skipping, short sprint bursts, or anything that expresses or adds to his joy in the activity.

A steady-state run means running a specified distance or length of time at a fairly even, comfortable pace. One of the objects of steady-state running is to increase the distance that can be covered smoothly and easily. The gradual increase in distance covered each week over 6 weeks or more builds strength, stamina, and self-confidence.

The schedules I make out for those I am advising generally include 1 day of each of these types of exercise on the 3 "hard" workout days of each week.

A typical schedule for a beginning jogger or rehabilitation patient who has completed at least 2 to 3 weeks of conditioning might look like this[1]:

MONDAY: Cover total distance of 1½ miles as follows:
1. Jog 110 yards, walk 110 yards.
2. Jog 220 yards, walk 220 yards.
3. Jog 110 yards, walk 110 yards.
4. Jog continuously but at varied pace (fartlek) for ¾ mile, including walking as needed.
5. Jog 110 yards, walk 110 yards.

TUESDAY: Walk 5 to 10 minutes; do easy stretching exercises.

WEDNESDAY: Cover total distance of 1½ miles as follows: Jog continuously for 1½ miles at as even a pace as possible, but slow to a walk occasionally if needed. The purpose of this exercise is to find the pace at which an individual can cover the distance at a steady-state run or jog and to develop the physical condition to do it easily. Improvement should be gradual.

THURSDAY: Walk 5 to 10 minutes; do easy stretching exercises.

FRIDAY: Cover total distance of 1½ miles as follows:
1. Jog 110 yards, walk 110 yards.
2. Jog 330 yards, walk 330 yards.
3. Jog slowly and steadily 880 yards. Walk as needed.
4. Jog 110 yards, walk 110 yards; repeat three times.

SATURDAY OR SUNDAY: Either walk 10 to 15 minutes or do stretching exercises, but not both.

REFERENCES

1. Bowerman, W.J., and Harris, W.E.: Jogging, New York, 1967, Grosset & Dunlap, Inc.
2. Lydiard, A.: Run to the top, Wellington, New Zealand, 1962, A.H. Reed & A.W. Reed, Ltd., Publishers.

5. Anatomy of a running shoe

William J. Bowerman

"In the beginning, God created the Heaven and the Earth. . . ." Having done this great thing, God probably recognized that he had also created a number of problems, one of which was man, who hastily went about producing problems of his own. Ever since Genesis, men have been seeking solutions to their problems, sometimes resolving them through divine guidance or other means, sometimes simply continuing to err in ways that try the patients of other men, their feet, and undoubtedly their Creator.

In the evolution of men, some become chiefs and the less fortunate became Indians. According to Boccaccio, one of the Arab chiefs, Abdul Ali Hassan, returned from a foray to the Persian Gulf and dismounting from his camel stepped on a thorn. He blasphemed for about 10 minutes and then issued a proclamation that all the earth should be covered with leather. His chief bearer, Muhamid Ali, was no fool and figured it would be easier to cover a foot than the world, even though Hassan would need a size $14^{1}/_{2}$. Was the Arabian peninsula and the area known as the Fertile Crescent therefore the home of the first shoe?

Not so, according to Luther Cressman, an anthropologist of some renown and a hunter of early *Homo sapiens* memorabilia. Cressman has presented evidence to the Oregon Museum of Natural History in Portland that man was shod as early as 10,000 years ago while living at a place now called Fort Rock in the high desert country of Oregon. One of the pre-Columbians left his shoes there, and about 10,000 years later Cressman came across them. No one has discovered an earlier shoe.

The descendants of pre-Columbian man, the Modoc Indians, made a simple shoe that we still call a moccasin. The vamp and tongue were one piece. The sole, heel, counter, and shank were another piece. The latch (lace or fastener) was threaded from counter to tongue. The entire shoe was made of leather and wonderfully simple (Fig. 5-1).

The original last was probably a foot-shaped river stone or a whittled chunk of hardwood. The modern last did not appear until the time of the Civil War. One last was used to make both a right and a left shoe.

To build a shoe one starts with the *last*. The last is a mold that looks somewhat like a foot and in the United States is graded according to men's sizes 5 to 13 (although it is possible to find or have lasts made in sizes 1 to 18). The average width for men's lasts is D, but they are made from widths AA (narrow) to EEE (wide). Lasts for women are generally $1^{1}/_{2}$ sizes smaller than for men: a women's size 7, for instance, is about the same length as a men's size $5^{1}/_{2}$. The average width for women is A, but widths run from AAA to EE. Infants' shoes run from sizes 1 to 13; children's shoes are made in a larger series of sizes 1 to 13. To further confuse the world, the European sizing system is metric, sizes 20 to 50, and the British system uses the same numbers as the American but each number designates about a full size larger.

Until a couple of years ago most shoes produced for joggers were made in a D width, but as the demand became greater and manufacturers more financially able, there were more variations to choose from, particularly for women. Unfortunately, the shoes began to look more like fashion shoes and less like feet.

The first step after choosing the last is to tack an *innersole* to the last. The innersole is cut from a pattern that almost exactly fits the bottom of the last.

The *upper* is the part of the shoe that is slipped over the top of the last and tacked at the toe, the heel around the Achilles tendon, and sometimes medially and laterally around the metatarsal heads (Fig. 5-2). In the standard running shoe the visible parts of the upper include the *vamp*, the part from the toe to midarch; the *quarter* from the vamp to the back of the heel; and *foxing*, which covers the seam at the center back of the heel. There is also the *vamp plug* (in moccasin-style shoes) or the *tongue*, which covers the upper part of the foot from the toes almost to the ankle. In laced shoes there are *eyelets* for the *latch* or laces. Eyelets have a *facing* that usually conceals reinforcing material to firm and prevent tearing out of the part of the quarter that contains the eyelets.

At the back or heel part of the upper is stitching that must be both strong and flexible. The stitching is strengthened and concealed either by a *backstay* or by the previously mentioned foxing, which has little use except to hide the stitching and trim the shoe.

An invisible but very important part of a shoe is the *heel counter*. It is concealed by the quarter, backstay, and foxing. It should give the heel stability, but if it is too stiff, it can cause bruises, blisters, or calluses. If too flexible or fragile, it is of no practical value. The real test of an acceptable heel counter will be passed when it satisfies multitudes of runners. Despite the scientific evaluations and advertising claims that have been made, no heel counter has yet passed this test.

The front part or vamp of a shoe may conceal a *toe box* made of the material used to strengthen and firm the vamp or made simply of the same material as the upper, as in moccasins. The toe box must provide adequate room for the mechanical function of the toes in running. Most manufacturers have given lip service to this requirement but actually have little or no knowledge of what happens from the metatarsal heads forward during running.

Several of the most common adaptations for uppers are (1) *standard*, which

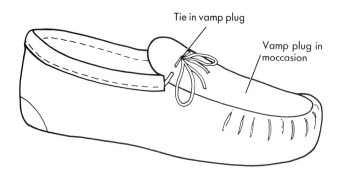

Fig. 5-1. Moccasin. Quarter, vamp, and sole are one piece. Backstay is rawhide.

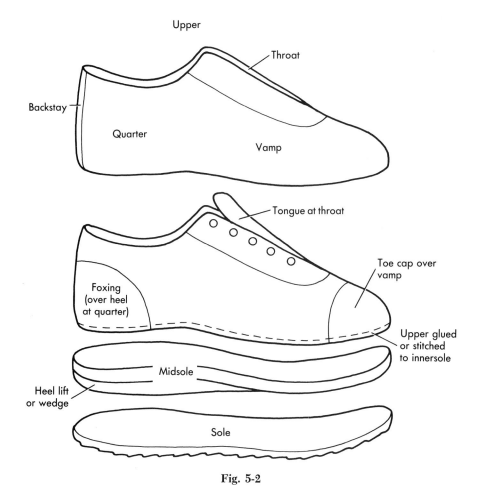

Fig. 5-2

includes vamp and quarters; (2) *moccasin*, which incorporates vamp and tongue; and (3) *slip lasted*, a California-designed upper that slips onto the last like a slipper.

The *midsole* and *heel wedge* for most running shoes are cemented together and then cut or "clicked" by a special machine to the appropriate size for cementing to the upper while it is tacked on to the last.

Finally, there is the *outsole*. The outsole usually is designed for traction (as in the waffle sole) and should be made of a long-wearing, nonskid compound. When this outsole is cemented to the midsole, the shoe is ready for its finishing treatment, which should include an appropriate amount of heat to allow the synthetic materials in the shoe to "memorize" the size the shoe is meant to be.

6. Hindfoot and midfoot problems of the runner

John F. Waller, Jr.

ANATOMY

Although this chapter deals with the hindfoot and midfoot, it is important to remember that the human body is a chain-linkage system. As a chain is made up of elliptical links connected by linkages, the human body is composed of bones connected by joints, which are stabilized directly by the ligaments and indirectly by the muscles attached to the bones or joints. A problem in any one of these segments can cause an imbalance in another segment, and the segment being affected secondarily may be more symptomatic than the primary site of involvement.

Hindfoot

The hindfoot is composed of the calcaneus and the talus. The calcaneus, constructed in a manner similar to a chicken's egg, has a tremendous ability to handle compression loads. The talus is the keystone of the foot. The subtalar joint allows inversion and eversion of the calcaneus on the talus and a simultaneous anterior and posterior rocking of the calcaneus on the talus. This movement has been likened to that of a corkscrew.[5] The subtalar joint acts as a torque converter, converting pronation and supination of the foot to internal and external rotatory forces in the leg. The subtalar joint is held together by talocalcaneal interosseous ligaments and secondarily by the deltoid ligament medially and the lateral ankle ligament complex laterally. Posteriorly, the triceps surae forms the Achilles tendon, which inserts approximately halfway down on the posterior aspect of the calcaneus. The upper portion of the calcaneus is separated from the Achilles tendon by a bursa. A second bursa separates the Achilles tendon from the skin and subcutaneous tissue. After its insertion onto the calcaneus, the Achilles tendon becomes thinner and broader, sweeps under the posteroinferior aspect of the heel, and projects forward as the plantar fascia after leaving the plantar medial and lateral tuberosities of the calcaneus. The plantar fascia projects anteriorly and inserts onto the sides of the metatarsal heads and, more important, onto the proximal phalanges of the toes.

64

Midfoot

The midfoot is composed of the navicular and cuboid bones and the three cuneiform bones. The midtarsal joint is bounded posteriorly by the talus and calcaneus and anteriorly by the navicular and cuboid bones. The varus and valgus swings of the calcaneus on the talus produce the relative locking and unlocking of the midtarsal joint.[1] The three cuneiform bones are bound to one another and the navicular and cuboid bones by strong ligaments that are rarely injured in the runner. The tibialis posterior muscle is the principal motor muscle acting on the midfoot. Its tendon inserts primarily onto the medial aspect of the navicular bone and secondarily onto the three cuneiform bones and the bases of the second, third, and fourth metatarsal heads.

HINDFOOT PROBLEMS

Most problems in the hindfoot and midfoot of the runner are related to multiple episodes of repeated microtrauma, which build up to cause pain and disability.

Plantar fasciitis—heel spur syndrome

The most common hindfoot problem in the runner is pain at the plantar surface of the calcaneus. Usually this pain is localized to the plantar medial tuberosity of the calcaneus where the plantar fascia takes origin. The pain is worse when the athlete first puts weight on the foot when getting out of bed in the morning, and it generally eases after a few steps or after a hot bath or shower. The runner commonly has a second episode of tenderness while cooling down after a long run. The athlete with this problem is usually more comfortable wearing a shoe with an elevated heel than walking barefoot or in a flat sandal.

This entity is believed to be a form of plantar fasciitis. The inflammation in the area of the origin of the plantar fascia results from excessive stress in the triceps surae, Achilles tendon, and plantar fascia linkage system (Fig. 6-1). The weak link is the origin of the plantar fascia, which is relatively narrow compared with the broad expansions and insertions of the plantar fascia onto the toes. An x-ray study may show an ossification of the origin of the plantar fascia, or no spur may be apparent. Many people without painful heels have this ossification present on x-ray studies. Pain is elicited when the area over the plantar medial tuberosity of the calcaneus is palpated. The gastroc-soleus—Achilles tendon complex is noted to be tight. This can be tested by passive and active dorsiflexon of the foot with the knee held in extension. If the foot cannot be placed in dorsiflexion of approximately 10 to 15 degrees beyond neutral, the posterior calf musculature is tight for a runner.

The treatment is vigorous stretching exercises for the calf muscles, which should be done at least three times a day. The runner is told to wear a shoe with a heel elevated at least $^1/_2$ to $^3/_4$ inch higher than the sole. If the pain is severe at the time of the initial visit, an orally administered anti-inflammatory agent may be given. The patient should be examined again in 3 weeks to make sure the stretching exercises are being done correctly. If the calf appears to be stretched and the pain

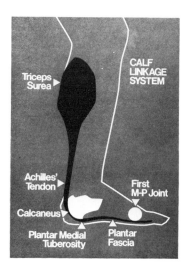

Fig. 6-1. Gastroc-soleus (calf) linkage system.

persists, one injection of corticosteroid may be tried. Another helpful adjunct in refractory cases is a shoe with a long rigid shank and a rocker sole. This reduces stress on the plantar fascia by limiting passive dorsiflexion of the toes during roll-off, thus negating or preventing the windlass action of the plantar fascia. Therefore the plantar fascia can be placed under less tension proximally by stretching the gastroc-soleus complex and distally by neutralizing the windlass action of the toes on the plantar fascia.[3]

Stress fracture of the calcaneus

A stress fracture of the calcaneus can also produce plantar calcaneal pain. Usually the patient has a sudden onset of pain, which is constant rather than the fluctuating pain occurring with plantar fasciitis. Medial and lateral compression of the tuberosity of the calcaneus usually causes severe pain. The initial x-ray examination does not reveal the presence of a fracture because the very thin cortex of the calcaneus does not show the break; it is usually 4 to 6 weeks before the sclerotic line that is a pathognomonic sign of the stress fracture appears (Fig. 6-2). Percussion tenderness is a good diagnostic sign of stress fracture. If this is present over the tuberosity of the calcaneus, a stress fracture should be assumed present until proved otherwise. A bone scan may be performed if the diagnosis is in doubt. The treatment is compressive dressings with rest, elevation, and range of motion exercises for the first 2 to 3 weeks. Weight-bearing in a running shoe to provide adequate cushioning is allowed as tolerated. Swimming is the best-tolerated sport to maintain aerobic power for runners with stress fractures. When percussion tenderness is gone and there is good subtalar motion, the runner may begin training again.

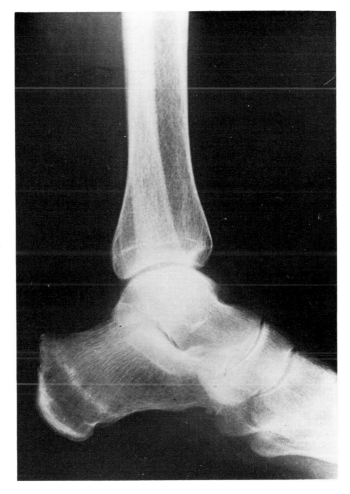

Fig. 6-2. Stress fracture of calcaneus.

Os trigonum syndrome

The os trigonum syndrome is a commonly missed pathologic condition in the hindfoot. The os trigonum is an accessory ossicle that in some individuals forms a synostosis with the posterior aspect of the talus. The os trigonum syndrome is manifested by pain in the back of the ankle during plantar flexion. The runner may feel this during roll-off on a flat surface or more acutely when running downhill. The mechanism of injury is usually plantar flexion and inversion stress that causes an initial sprain of the lateral ankle ligament complex. After the ligaments are healed and the foot and leg are rehabilitated, there is persistence of pain behind the ankle during plantar flexion. The examiner can elicit pain with forced plantar flexion of the foot. X-ray studies reveal the presence of an os trigonum separated from the talus by a vertical lucent line (Fig. 6-3). It is difficult to tell whether the patient has

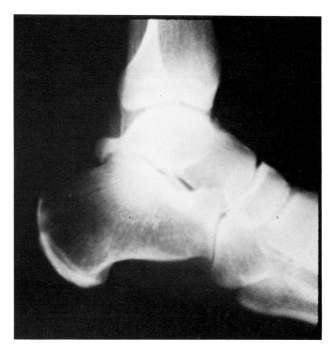

Fig. 6-3. Os trigonum.

had long-standing pseudarthrosis of the os trigonum or whether a synostosis or syndesmosis has been disrupted. Apparently the latter occurs when the os trigonum is caught between the posterior aspect of the distal tibia and the superior surface of the calcaneus. The only effective treatment is excision of the os trigonum, after which most runners can return to training in approximately 3 weeks.

Retroachilles and retrocalcaneal bursitis

Pain over the posterosuperior lateral prominence of the calcaneus is commonly referred to as the pump-bump syndrome because it often occurs in women who wear high-heeled shoes. There are two bursae in this area. One lies between the subcutaneous tissue and the Achilles tendon and the other between the Achilles tendon and the calcaneus. (Note that there are far fewer bursae in the foot than there are areas of bursitis diagnosed and treated with injection.) This is one of the few entities in which marked inflammation can lead to complete degeneration of the bursa between the Achilles tendon and the calcaneus. The pain in a pump-bump syndrome is not related directly to the size and shape of the bump, as Haglund has suggested. Many people with large protuberant heels have no pain at all. Others, who have a normal-appearing calcaneus, have severe pain over the postero-superior lateral prominence of the calcaneus. However, individuals who have a prominent calcaneus may have a predisposition to degeneration of the retrocalcaneal bursa.

The initial treatment is removal of pressure from the posterior aspect of the calcaneus. This can be done in one of three ways: the heel counter of the shoe can be lowered, the patient can wear a clog, or an orthotist can build a heel cup that will relieve stress in the affected area. If the retrocalcaneal bursa is severely inflamed or swollen, it may be evacuated. If pain persists despite these treatments, surgical exploration should be performed. I have not found bursal remnants during surgery, and therefore I believe the pain is caused by the tendon being pushed directly against the bony prominence of the calcaneus. The calcaneus should be excised from the insertion of the Achilles tendon superiorly. The bursa between the skin and the Achilles tendon can also become inflamed. This usually happens when the runner is wearing a shoe in which the heel counter is too large. The dorsal extension of the heel counter rubs against the back of the heel, causing inflammation and swelling in the retroachilles bursa. This is treated with an open-back shoe or clog, a 5-day course of an anti-inflammatory drug to reduce the inflammation, the use of warm soaks, and if necessary an aspiration of the bursa.

MIDFOOT PROBLEMS
Posterior tibialis tendinitis

The posterior tibial tendon at its insertion onto the navicular bone may be the site of severe pain in the runner. The pain commonly occurs after a twisting injury to the foot. After the immediate symptoms of the injury resolve, the runner is left with persistent pain over the medial aspect of the foot. Most patients with this symptom complex have a palpable prominence, which is reflected as an accessory navicular bone on x-ray study (Fig. 6-4). The treatment is rest of the posterior tibial tendon. A ⅛-inch inner heel lift with an additional ⅛-inch inner heel wedge should be inserted in the shoe. This should be augmented with a vigorous stretching program for the posterior calf muscles and a gentle, progressive, power exercise program for the tibialis posterior muscle. If the pain persists after 6 weeks, an oral anti-inflammatory drug should be given and a temporary orthotic should be considered. Few patients require surgical revision of the insertion of the posterior tibial tendon onto the navicular bone. I have not observed pain referable to the peroneal tendons in the hindfoot and midfoot in patients who have good subtalar motion and have not had fractures of the calcaneus.

Anterolateral corner compression syndrome of the foot

The anterolateral corner compression syndrome is pain referable to the antero-inferior border of the fibula and the anterolateral surface of the talus. The patient may instead complain of pain in the anterolateral corner of the foot or at the insertion of the posterior tibial tendon on the navicular bone. Symptoms of pain may occur in all three areas. The runner usually has a history of numerous inversion injuries that occur even though there are no gross deformities in the running surface. A physical examination shows a heel valgus alignment with some pronation of the subtalar joint and an associated descent of the arch. Pain can be elicited by

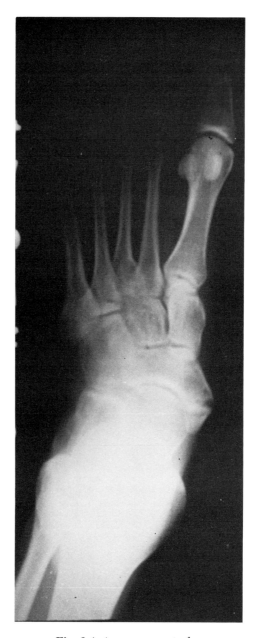

Fig. 6-4. Accessory navicular.

deep palpation of the area between the anteroinferior border of the fibula and the anterolateral portion of the talus. When questioned, the patient commonly states that he attempts to hold his feet in an inverted position for comfort. X-ray studies of the foot and ankle show no abnormalities. I believe this entity to be a synovial compression syndrome or a chondromalacia of the lateral wall of the dome of the talus. To relieve the talofibular compression syndrome, the patient tightens the posterior tibial tendon and relaxes the peroneal tendons, making him susceptible to repeated inversion injuries. When the compression is released, the posterior tibial and peroneal tendons are again balanced and the inversion injuries cease. It is important to be aware of this disorder because the pain may be referred and the primary area of involvement should not be missed. The treatment is to apply a $^1/_8$- to $^3/_{16}$-inch inner heel and inner sole wedge to the shoes. With the use of the wedge, the pain usually disappears within a few days and the inversion injuries stop. I have also found a ready-made orthotic, the Lynco Biomechanical Support, to be of great help.

Tarsal tunnel syndrome

The tarsal tunnel syndrome is relatively rare, especially in the runner. It is commonly manifested by severe forefoot pain. The posterior tibial nerve enters the foot through a fibrous tunnel in the flexor retinaculum. In the foot the nerve splits into three branches. The first branch to leave the main trunk is the medial calcaneal nerve, a sensory branch that may split from the main trunk proximal to the flexor retinaculum. The medial plantar and lateral plantar nerves are mixed nerves that branch off in the distal portion of the posterior tibial nerve, usually in the body of the abductor hallucis muscle. Compression of the nerve in the laciniate ligament or in the body of the abductor hallucis muscle causes pain and paresthesias in the forefoot. When an individual with a markedly pronated foot wears a shoe with a hard scaphoid pad, the posterior tibial nerve or one of its two distal branches can become compressed, causing a tarsal tunnel–like syndrome. This is usually a neurapraxia and clears in 4 to 6 weeks after the scaphoid pad has been removed from the shoe. In patients with tarsal tunnel syndrome a Tinel's sign can be elicited over the area of compression.[4] The initial therapy should be a medial heel wedge to put the heel in a more neutral or slightly varus position. This helps reduce the tension on the neurovascular bundle in the laciniate ligament. The treatment can be augmented with the use of anti-inflammatory drugs. The shoes should be checked for possible areas of compression against the nerves. Conduction studies should be performed, although they may show no definite evidence of nerve damage. If rest and balancing the foot do not help, surgical decompression of the posterior tibial nerve in the laciniate ligament and the abductor hallucis muscle should be performed.

LIGAMENTOUS INTEGRITY IN THE HINDFOOT AND MIDFOOT

The ligamentous integrity of the subtalar and midtarsal joints has a profound effect on the shape and biomechanics of the foot. An individual with a pronated foot has a heel valgus alignment, a descent of the arch, an abducted forefoot, and a medial prominence in the area of the midfoot corresponding to a medial subluxation of the talonavicular joint. This is often a reflection of ligamentous laxity not only in the subtalar joint but also in the midtarsal and cuneonavicular joints. A foot of this type is very supple and is referred to as a flexible flatfoot. The flexible flatfoot is often blamed for problems elsewhere in the human linkage system. It should not be viewed as a pathological condition unless there is severe deformity or symptoms related specifically to the subtalar or midtarsal joints. A relative ligamentous laxity with some descent of the arch and heel valgus alignment is necessary for the runner because it provides springiness and cushioning in the foot and ankle complex during heel strike and midstance. It also adapts better to the running surface than a foot with a higher arch·and less flexibility. The most common problem associated with flexible flatfoot is the coexistence of a tight gastroc-soleus complex, which was first documented by Harris and Beath.[2] The patient may also have a relative weakness of the plantar flexors and invertors and dorsiflexors and evertors. I believe it is necessary to balance the musculature controlling the foot, ankle, and leg before resorting to an orthotic to balance the foot.

When the ligaments in the midfoot and the hindfoot are very stiff, the foot usually takes on a high arch or cavus-type conformation. This type of foot causes problems in its inability to help absorb shock and provide springiness and cushioning to the foot and proximal linkage system. Also, it does not accommodate easily to different running surfaces. Pain develops under the metatarsals and in the heel, and breakdown occurs in the more proximal portions of the linkage system as a result of overloading. The best way to handle these problems is vigorous stretching exercises to allow the runner to land farther back on the heel, providing a more rolling motion in the foot and ankle complexes during the stance phase of gait. A shoe with extra cushioning is also necessary.

SUMMARY

Most problems of the hindfoot and midfoot are related to repeated episodes of microtrauma and are referred to as overuse syndromes. The pathological condition can usually be analyzed in terms of the defect in the use or balance of the human linkage system. With proper muscle balancing, the use of a shoe that provides cushioning, and in some cases support with a wedge or an orthotic, most problems in the hindfoot and midfoot of the runner can be easily resolved.

REFERENCES

1. Elftman, H.: The transverse tarsal joint and its control, Clin. Orthop. **16**:41, 1960.
2. Harris, R.I., and Beath, T.: Hypermobile flat-foot with short tendo Achillis, J. Bone Joint Surg. **30A**:116, 1948.
3. Hicks, J.H.: The mechanics of the foot. II. The plantar aponeurosis and the arch, Arch. J. Anat. **88**:25, 1954.
4. Mann, R.A.: Tarsal tunnel syndrome, Orthop. Clin. North Am. **5**:109, 1974.
5. Manter, J.T.: Movements of the subtalar and transverse tarsal joints, Anat. Rec. **80**:397, 1941.

7. Forefoot problems in runners

David Drez, Jr.

Pain beneath the forefoot has been defined as metatarsalgia. This is an imprecise term, and the disorder was clarified by Scranton, who analyzed a series of patients with pain in the forepart of the foot and grouped their diagnoses under three main headings:

1. Primary metatarsalgia
2. Secondary metatarsalgia
3. Symptoms of pain under the forepart of the foot unrelated to disorders in weight distribution across the metatarsal articulation

Patients with primary metatarsalgia had pain across the metatarsophalangeal joint articulation with reactive plantar keratoses. An imbalance in weight distribution between the toes and the metatarsal heads was present. This group included such conditions as hallux valgus, metatarsal pain following bunionectomy, hallux rigidus, and Freiberg's disease.

Secondary metatarsalgia was caused by metatarsophalangeal joint imbalance from influences other than the metatarsals. Included under this heading were systemic diseases such as rheumatoid arthritis and gout, as well as metatarsal stress fractures and sesamoid abnormalities.

The third group was those with forefoot pain unrelated to disorders of weight distribution across the metatarsophalangeal joint articulation. Included in this group were such conditions as Morton's neuroma, plantar fasciitis, tarsal tunnel syndrome, and plantar warts.

This chapter deals with problems of the forefoot that I have seen at the Runner's Clinic at Louisiana State University in New Orleans. A list of suggested readings appears at the end of the chapter for those who wish to pursue certain aspects in more detail.

Calluses are reactive keratotic masses occurring commonly in the feet of runners. If the calluses are symptomatic, treatment to distribute weight-bearing forces more evenly is needed. Total-contact molded inserts constructed of Plastizote #2 alone or covered by a closed-cell neoprene material have been used. The neoprene material may also be used alone.

Freiberg's infraction or osteochondrosis of the metatarsal head is probably the result of a vascular insult to the primary growth center of the metatarsal head. The second metatarsal is usually involved. This condition commonly appears in the second decade of life. Tenderness and pain localized to the involved metatarsal head are present. Pads are used to relieve pressure. If this fails, an arthroplasty of the involved joint to reshape the metatarsal head and remove loose fragments may be effective. Metatarsal head excision should be avoided.

The treatment of symptomatic *hallux valgus* in the runner should consist primarily of nonoperative measures. Since the patient usually has some degree of excessive pronation, use of an arch support and widening the running shoe over the prominence offer success in many cases. Patients unresponsive to such treatment may require an operative procedure to correct the varus deformity of the first metatarsal and a soft tissue procedure to tighten the medial capsule of the metatarsophalangeal joint.

Hallux rigidus is a disabling condition in the runner. Dorsiflexion of the metatarsophalangeal joint of the great toe is limited and painful. Bony proliferation around the joint usually involves only the dorsal surface. Operative treatment by excision of the proliferative bone dorsally (cheilectomy) has been successful in the few cases in which I have used it.

Corns are seen commonly over the lateral aspect of the proximal interphalangeal joint of the fifth toe in the runner. Initially the patient is treated nonoperatively with the use of doughnut-type pads. Operative removal of the prominent exostosis beneath the reactive corn is easily performed and very successful.

A *mallet toe* in which there is flexion of the distal phalanx on the middle phalanx may result in significant pain over the distal aspect of the toe in a runner. If shoe modification and cushioning fail to alleviate symptoms, the head of the middle phalanx can be excised.

A *hammer toe deformity* in which there is flexion of the middle and distal phalanx on the proximal phalanx may produce a painful corn over the dorsal aspect of the proximal interphalangeal joint, resulting in significant discomfort to the runner. If shoe modification and padding fail to alleviate symptoms, operative treatment should be employed. Arthrodesis of the proximal interphalangeal joint is usually performed in the runner under 35 years of age. Excision of the proximal half of the proximal phalanx is recommended for the older patient.

Sesamoiditis and *stress fractures of the sesamoids* are not uncommon causes of pain in the runner. If symptoms fail to resolve after nonoperative treatment with pads and cushioning, excision of the involved sesamoid may be necessary.

Stress fractures of the metatarsals are common injuries. The short first metatarsal or Morton's toe is not a cause of metatarsal stress fractures. The treatment consists of activity modification with resumption of activity as pain allows.

Interdigital neuroma is more common in female runners. The treatment is pads and corticosteroid injection. Excision of the neuroma in cases unresponsive to these measures usually results in permanent relief of symptoms.

Plantar warts are extremely painful lesions in runners. I have used the treatment technique popularized by Dr. William F. Wagner of Whittier, California. A 1% plain lidocaine solution is injected directly beneath the wart so that a small bleb is raised and blanching of the skin occurs. Up to nine injections may be needed to effect a cure. The wart falls off, and no residual scar is left.

The runner with an *ingrown toenail* usually seeks treatment when infection is present and pain makes running impossible. Initial treatment to control the infection is necessary. Complete nail removal is not recommended. Instead, the nail margin is removed with the patient under local anesthesia. If both sides of the nail are involved, both nail margins are removed, leaving the central portion of the nail in place. If complete cure is not achieved and the condition recurs, the nail margin, matrix, and nail groove are excised.

Blisters result from shear stress and may be prevented by applying petroleum jelly to the feet. An established painful blister may be treated by unroofing the blister under sterile conditions and covering its base with Betadine Ointment. The symptoms are relieved, and the patient can rapidly return to competition.

Subungual hematoma (black toe) is caused by trauma to the end of the toe by the shoe. This condition may be painful, but it is of little importance and should be ignored in most cases.

SUGGESTED READINGS

Drez, D., Jr.: Current orthopaedic management, Edinburgh, 1981, Churchill Livingstone.

Drez, D., Jr., and others: Metatarsal stress fractures, Am. J. Sports Med. **8:**123, 1980.

Giannestras, N.J.: Foot disorders: medical and surgical management, ed. 2, Philadelphia, 1973, Lea & Febiger.

Mann, R.A.: DuVries' surgery of the foot, ed. 4, St. Louis, 1978, The C.V. Mosby Co.

Mann, R.A., and others: Running symposium, Foot Ankle **1:**199, 1981.

Scranton, P.E., Jr.: Metatarsalgia: diagnosis and treatment, J. Bone Joint Surg. **62A:**723, 1980.

Scranton, P.E., Jr.: Metatarsalgia: a clinical review of diagnosis and management, Foot Ankle **1:**229, 1981.

Scranton, P.E., Jr., and Rutkowski, R.: Anatomic variations in the first ray, Clin. Orthop. **151:**256, 1980.

8. Orthotics and shoe corrections*

Dennis E. Vixie

Because of the boom in athletic activity and the national desire for people to keep fit, we orthotists now have to deal with minute misalignment problems as well as the more usual orthotic management problems. Running has become one of the most popular of all athletic activities. Most of the population is unaware of the importance of proper training and equipment for this sport. People of all ages and in all events, from sprinters and distance runners to hurdlers, have suffered running injuries.

When referring a patient to an orthotist, the physician describes the malady or injury, and it is the orthotist's task to design, manufacture, and fit a corrective or supportive orthotic or shoe modification. The steps the orthotist takes for this are as follows:

1. Evaluating the shoe for the sport or activity in which the patient is engaged, in this case running or jogging
2. Evaluating the patient's feet and body alignment to determine if there is a misalignment that was not perceived in the original evaluation by the physician

Orthotists go through the steps listed below to determine the proper footwear for the patient. This evaluation prevents many of the small injuries that occur when the runner does not wear the proper shoe or a good-quality shoe made for running.

1. Check that the shoe is built for running with good heel and forefoot cushioning.
2. Determine that the last is proper for the patient's foot type—a straight last for a patient with a normal or flexible foot or a combination last for a patient with a semirigid or rigid foot (Fig. 8-1). This is done by mentally bisecting the heel and drawing a line of progression to determine if the design of the last is in valgus or varus alignment.
3. Determine the rigidity of the heel counter by squeezing the posterior section

---

*Orthotics is a rapidly changing field, and this chapter presents only a brief overview. Questions on this subject may be directed to the author of the chapter.

of the shoe. The shoe must reduce the amount of pronation to keep the foot in its normal range of motion. The shoes on the market today are very marginal in this regard, but a shoe with a fairly rigid counter can be obtained.

4. Make sure the patient has a snug fit in the heel to control the shoe properly. A heel that is not snugly fitted encourages pronation of the foot (Fig. 8-2). Check that there is room in the forefoot for the foot to splay out during the stance phase.

5. Check that the shoe has the proper alignment in the heel. A straight foundation is necessary. Because the larger shoe companies are more automated and there is less chance of human error, their products have a more reliable alignment. As in Fig. 8-3, check that the heel being bisected is perpendicular to the ground. A shoe built in pronation (Fig. 8-3, *A*) forces the runner into pronation. If the shoe is built in supination, it causes excessive wear on the lateral part of the heel and the runner cannot achieve the required toe-off position (Fig. 8-3, *B*). Even if the shoe has a factory heel wedge, the heel should be perpendicular. If the sole is lasted off center, the extra leverage can cause excessive pronation (Fig. 8-3, *C*) or supination (Fig. 8-3, *D*).

After the shoe is evaluated, the following patient evaluation is the next procedure:

1. First check the patient standing with feet 1 inch apart to see if the feet are in valgus or varus alignment.

2. Have the patient lie prone on an examining table with the feet extended over the edge 1 inch apart. Mentally bisect the calf and the heel at the insertion of the Achilles tendon, and then push up on the foot joint behind the fifth metatarsal head with the talus in neutral position just until you feel resistance. The back of the calf and heel should be in line. While the patient is prone with the foot relaxed, by bisecting the calf and the insertion of the Achilles tendon you can measure with the goniometer to determine if the heel alignment is valgus or varus.

If the patient has a fairly normal or slightly limited range of motion, a cast is applied by wrapping plaster splints on the patient's foot along the plantar surface and on the medial side to the navicular bone, around the heel to these two marks, and then around the toes so that the cast can be easily removed. The foot is pushed up behind the fifth metatarsal head as in the evaluation and the talus is kept in a neutral position until the plaster dries. From this cast a positive mold is made for the manufacture of the orthotic.

The orthotic built from the mold can be either soft or hard. A soft orthotic is all that is needed in 60% to 80% of the patients. The hard orthotic is produced from the same mold as the soft but is made of nylon acrylic, which gives more support across the plantar fascia. A hard orthotic can also be made by stiffening the soft orthotic with a hardening material. These orthotics can be obtained from an orthotic and prosthetic laboratory or a podiatry laboratory.

If the physician's evaluation shows that the patient needs a special shoe, it is

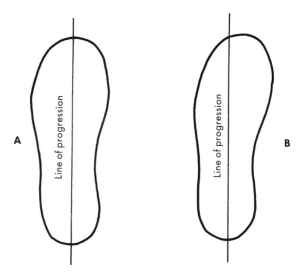

Fig. 8-1. **A,** Straight last for normal or very flexible foot. **B,** Combination last for semiridged and supinated foot.

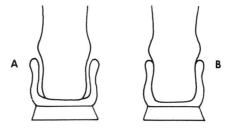

Fig. 8-2. **A,** Less-than-snug fit allows pronation in shoe. **B,** Snug fit allows wearer to control shoe.

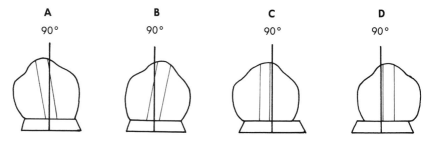

Fig. 8-3. **A,** Lasted in pronation. **B,** Lasted in supination. **C,** Sole lasted off center to lateral side. **D,** Sole lasted off center to medial side.

built by casting the patient's foot as in the casting procedure previously described, except that the whole foot is wrapped to 1 inch above the malleolus. A special shoe is usually necessary when a patient has an abnormally flexible or rigid foot for which the normal leverage must be produced by the shoe. The first step in making a special shoe is to make a positive mold from the cast taken of the patient's foot. The mold is modified to be snug in the heel and roomy in the forefoot. From the modified mold a last is made. An upper is made or a premade upper is modified to create the leverages needed to prevent the problem. The upper is then glued to the midsole, which is attached to the last, and pulled into place, and then the sole is applied in the appropriate alignment for the leverages required. The shoe is then complete.

Custom-made shoes can eliminate or reduce many problems that cannot be controlled with orthotics. Unfortunately, it is hard to find someone willing to build the specific shoes needed. Another problem is the cost to the patient, $200 and up depending on the area of the United States. Only 2% to 3% of the patients referred to us have needed special shoes.

9. Muscle and tendon physiology

Ejnar Eriksson
Tom Häggmark

MOTOR UNIT

When a human muscle performs work, it is one part in a system composed of an alpha motor neuron in the spinal cord and a motor nerve that connects the neuron with the appropriate muscle fibers. Although there are different types of muscle fiber, all the fibers connected to a given motor neuron in the spinal cord have the same properties and are of the same type.[6] The alpha motor neuron, motor nerve, and muscle fibers together make up the motor unit, the basic functional unit in the skeletal muscle system. It is the smallest part that can be activated, and it functions according to the "all-or-nothing law," which means that it is either fully activated or not activated at all. Each motor unit contains a varying number of muscle fibers depending on the type of muscle. In the finger muscles the motor units contain very few fibers, whereas in the leg muscles a motor unit can contain 200 to 800 fibers.[5]

MUSCLE FIBERS

Human skeletal muscle is composed of different kinds of motor units in which the connected muscle fibers have different properties. One of the functional differences between the muscle fibers is the speed of contraction. In vivo microelectrode stimulation produces a relatively short time to peak tension (about 30 msec) in the white muscle or fast twitch fibers. The other main group of fibers, the red muscle or slow twitch fibers, has a longer time to peak tension (about 90 msec) (Fig. 9-1).[3,4] The contractile properties of the muscle fibers can be evaluated by a histochemical method in which the activity of the enzyme myosin adenosinetriphosphatase (ATPase) is analyzed at different pH values.[2]

Another difference between the two main types of muscle fibers is that the type I or slow twitch fibers have a high capacity for oxidative metabolism and a greater ability to oxidize fat and produce energy. Thus they have a great endurance capacity. They are also surrounded by relatively more capillaries than the fast twitch fibers, and their fiber area is somewhat smaller than that of the fast twitch fibers

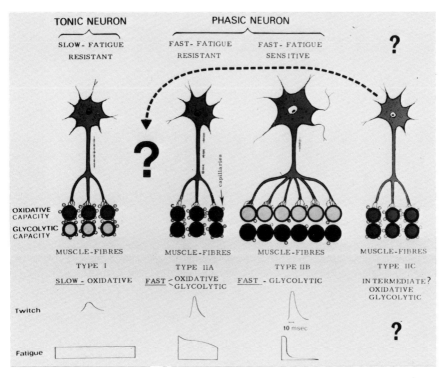

Fig. 9-1. Types and characteristics of muscle fibers and motor neurons. (Reprinted with permission from Eriksson, Ejnar, M.D., 1980. Muscle physiology: adaptation of the musculoskeletal system to exercise. Contemporary Orthopaedics **2**[3]:228-232. Courtesy of Bobit Publishing Co.)

(Fig. 9-1). In a training program such as jogging in which mainly the slow twitch fibers are activated, their oxidative capacity increases considerably, the volume of mitochondriae within the cells increases, and the activity of the oxidative enzymes increases. The number of capillaries around the muscle fibers also increases while the fiber area remains largely unchanged (Fig. 9-2).

The type II or fast twitch fibers have a short time of contraction. These fibers are divided into subgroups on the basis of their metabolic patterns. The main groups are IIA and IIB or FTA and FTB (fast twitch A and fast twitch B). The type IIB fiber has a high glycolytic capacity and a very short time to peak tension, and it can develop more power than the type I fiber. It is, however, rapidly fatigued and can work for only a short period. There is much evidence that these fibers are activated in movements, such as weight-lifting, in which a rapid muscle tension development is necessary. The energy in the fiber is produced by splitting glycogen in anaerobic glycolysis to produce adenosine triphosphate (ATP) and lactate. The type IIB fibers have a low oxidative capacity and are also surrounded by relatively few capillaries, but they contain more contractile protein than the type I fibers and have a larger cross-sectional area (Fig. 9-1). During a training program the glycol-

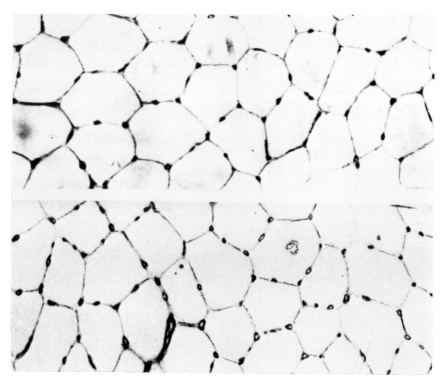

Fig. 9-2. Special staining for capillaries. Subject was cross-country skier before *(upper)* and after *(lower)* 6-week training period. Significant increase in number of capillaries occurred. (Courtesy of P. Schantz.)

ytic capacity increases considerably and the fiber area also increases, reflecting the increase of contractile proteins. The oxidative capacity remains on the same level.

Type IIA fibers have intermediate properties between the type I and type IIB fiber groups. Type IIA has higher glycolytic capacity than type I but not quite as high as type IIB. It has a higher oxidative capacity than type IIB but not as high as type I. Its number of capillaries is increased during training, and it has a somewhat larger fiber area than type I and type IIB, although the fiber area does not increase during training (Fig. 9-2).

It has recently been suggested that there is also a type IIC fiber that is intermediate between type I and type IIB.

EFFECT OF TRAINING ON MUSCLE FIBERS

Thanks to the technique of percutaneous muscle biopsy popularized by Bergström[1] in Sweden, many physiological studies of the effects of different kinds of training on muscle fibers have been performed. These studies have provided a basic understanding of the changes in the muscle after training, but they have also

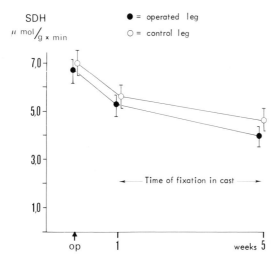

Fig. 9-3. One week after knee ligament reconstruction, oxidative activity measured by succinic dehydrogenase (SDH) has already fallen dramatically. (From Eriksson, E., and Häggmark, T.: Syntex Terapi **2**:92, 1977.)

revealed the complexity of the muscle mechanism. It seems that in most movements in everyday life the type I or slow twitch fibers are activated. These fibers also show the greatest changes after endurance training. Their aerobic metabolic capacity increases; that is, the mitochondriae occupy a greater area of the muscle fibers, the oxidative enzyme activity increases, and the capillary net is increased so that oxygen can easily be transported to the muscle cells. There is, however, no demand for an increase in the amount of contractile proteins, and the cell area is therefore not affected. The increase in oxidative capacity is also seen in the type II fibers but is less pronounced than in the type I fibers. The training of heavy weight-lifting, in which a maximum tension development in a very short time is needed, affects mainly the type II fibers. In this case there is an increase in the amount of contractile proteins and the myosin-actin filaments in the type II fibers, increasing the fiber area and the cross-sectional area of the total muscle.[8]

None of the studies has shown great changes in the proportions of type I and type II fibers following training. Within the type II group, however, there seem to be increases in the number of type IIA fibers after physical training.[11] It is known that with certain diseases and after injuries and immobilization there is a change of muscle fiber types.[7] It is also evident that the changes seen in skeletal muscle after training are relatively short lived if training is not continued. After immobilization of an extremity in a plaster cast the oxidative capacity drops significantly in 1 week (Fig. 9-3).[10]

The depletion of glycogen from different types of fibers after different types of activities has been widely investigated. These studies show that most types of activities involve the type I and type IIA fibers. Only in activities requiring rapid development of muscle tension are the type IIB fibers used.

BIOMECHANICAL PROPERTIES OF MUSCLES AND TENDONS

The biomechanical strength of muscles and tendons is proportional to their transverse areas. A tendon in humans has a strength of about 60 newtons/mm^2, whereas skeletal muscle has been found to have a strength of only 0.3 newton/mm^2 according to Yamada.[17] The significance of these figures is questionable, however, since they were extrapolated from experiments made 2 days after death. In the functional clinical unit of bone, tendon, and muscle, the tendon and muscle have approximately equal strength when tested immediately after death.[15] Yamada's figures for muscle strength should mean that the cross-sectional area of the muscle is about 200 times that of its tendon. The fascia surrounding the muscle is also believed to play a significant role in muscle strength.[16] When muscles are immobilized, they lose some of their tensile properties.[12] Within 1 week the breaking strength decreases by 20%, and within 3 weeks it falls further to about 70% of the normal breaking strength. Thus injured muscles heal faster if mobilized.[12-14]

Muscle size has often been determined by measuring the circumference of an

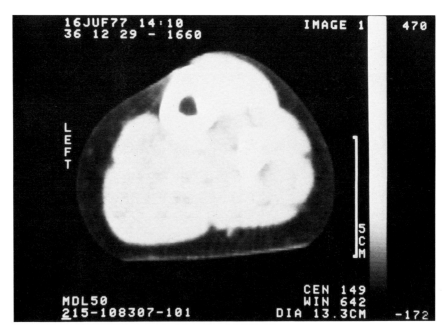

Fig. 9-4. Computed tomogram of calf of patient treated surgically for Achilles tendon rupture 6 weeks earlier. Significant atrophy of gastrocnemius and soleus muscles has occurred, but concomitant increase in subcutaneous space has also taken place so that measurement of circumference does not reveal true degree of atrophy.

extremity.[7] This is a relatively poor method of measurement, since muscle atrophy often is accompanied by an increase of the subcutaneous tissues. Thus a measurement of the circumference does not reveal the true degree of muscle atrophy.[9] Ultrasonography and computed tomography are more reliable methods of measurement (Fig. 9-4).[9]

REFERENCES

1. Bergström, J.: Muscle electrolytes in man, Scand. J. Clin. Lab. Invest. **14**(suppl. 68):1, 1962.
2. Brooke, M.H., and Kaiser, K.K.: Muscle fiber types: how many and what kind? Arch. Neurol. **23**:369, 1970.
3. Buchthal, F., and Schmalbruch, H.: Contraction times and fiber types in intact human muscle, Acta Physiol. Scand. **79**:435, 1970.
4. Buchthal, F., Dahl, K., and Rosenfalch, P.: Rise time of the spike potential in fast and slowly contracting muscle of man, Acta Physiol. Scand. **87**:261, 1973.
5. Burke, R.D., and others: Physiological types and histochemical profiles in motor units of the cat gastrocnemius, J. Physiol. **234**:723, 1973.
6. Edström, L., and Kugelberg, E.: Histochemical composition, distribution of fibres and fatiguability of single motor units, J. Neurol. Neurosurg. Pshychiatry **31**:424, 1968.
7. Eriksson, E.: Muscle physiology: adaptation of the muscular skeletal system to exercise, Contemp. Orthop. **2**:228, 1980.
8. Gollnick, P.D., and others: Enzyme activity and fiber composition in skeletal muscle of untrained and trained men, J. Appl. Physiol. **33**:312, 1972.
9. Häggmark, T., and Eriksson, E.: Hypotrophy of the soleus muscle in man after Achilles tendon rupture: discussion of findings obtained by computed tomography and morphologic studies, Am. J. Sports Med. **7**:121, 1979.
10. Häggmark, T., Jansson, E., and Eriksson, E.: Fiber type area and metabolic potential of the thigh muscle after knee surgery and immobilisation, Int. J. Sports Med. **2**:12, 1981.
11. Jansson, E., Sjödin, B., and Tesch, P.: Changes in muscle fiber type distribution in men after physical training, Acta Physiol. Scand. **104**:235, 1978.
12. Järvinen, M.: Healing of a crush injury in rat striated muscle, Academic thesis, Medical Faculty of the University of Turku, Turku, Finland, 1976.
13. Laros, G.S., Tipton, C.M., and Cooper, R.R.: Influence of physical activity on ligament insertions in the knees of dogs, J. Bone Joint Surg. **53A**:275, 1971.
14. Noyes, F.R., De Lucas, J.L., and Torvik, P.J.: Biomechanics of anterior cruciate ligament failure: an analysis of strain-rate sensitivity and mechanisms of failure in primates, J. Bone Joint Surg. **56A**:236, 1974.
15. Viidik, A.: Tensile strength properties of Achilles tendon systems in trained and untrained rabbits, Acta Orthop. Scand. **40**:261, 1969.
16. Viidik, A.: Elastomechanik biologischer Gewebe (Elastomechanics of biological tissues). In Kotta, H., Krahl, H., and Steinbrück, K., editors: Die Belastungstoleranz des Bewegungsapparates, Stuttgart, 1980, Thieme-Stratton, Inc.
17. Yamada, H.: Strength of biological materials, Baltimore, 1970, The Williams & Wilkins Co.

10. Biomechanics and rehabilitation of the gastroc-soleus complex

John F. Waller, Jr.

ANATOMY

The two heads of the gastrocnemius muscle have their origin at the medial and lateral femoral condyles of the knee. The soleus muscle has its origin at the proximal tibia and fibula. The two muscles coalesce to form the Achilles tendon, which inserts approximately halfway down on the posterior surface of the calcaneus. After attaching to the calcaneus, the Achilles tendon forms a fixed band that continues under the plantar aspect of the heel and projects forward as the plantar fascia. The Achilles tendon becomes the plantar fascia after leaving the plantar medial and plantar lateral tuberosities of the calcaneus. The plantar fascia extends anteriorly as bands that diverge and insert onto the medial and lateral aspects of the metatarsal heads and, more important, onto the proximal phalanges of the toes. It is this insertion onto the proximal phalanges of the toes that permits the "windlass action" of the plantar fascia.[1]

BIOMECHANICS

During ambulation the gastroc-soleus or triceps surae muscle complex can act in one of three ways: (1) the muscle can shorten and develop tension (concentric contraction); (2) the muscle can develop tension as it is being stretched (eccentric contraction); or (3) the muscle can tighten with no change in length (isometric contraction). The gastroc-soleus complex functions principally during the stance phase of gait, which may be broken down into two segments: heel strike to midstance and midstance to roll-off. During the first segment the foot is "unlocked" and the plantar fascia is relaxed so that the foot can accommodate to the surface being walked on or run on. During the second segment, the foot undergoes a locking that involves an alteration in the subtalar and midtarsal joints, as well as an activation and tightening of the plantar fascia. This allows the flexible foot to become a more rigid structure suitable for supporting the body during forward motion. These mechanisms, as well as control of the knee and upper body, depend on the function of the gastroc-soleus complex.

86

When an individual goes from a quiet stance position to toe standing, which involves a concentric contraction of the gastroc-soleus complex, the Achilles tendon exerts a symmetrical pull on the calcaneus. The varus and valgus rocking of the calcaneus on the talus is mediated by the shape of the subtalar joint and not by an asymmetrical pull of the calf muscles on the calcaneus.[2] Tension is created in the plantar fascia as the calf muscle tenses because the plantar fascia is a direct extension of the Achilles tendon. Tension also develops in the plantar fascia as a result of the windlass mechanism during the roll-off phase of gait.

The muscles of propulsion in the runner are those in the low back and in and around the hip. The principal function of the quadriceps muscles, hamstrings, calf muscles, and anterior tibial muscles is to control the motions of the thigh, leg, and foot during the stance and swing phases of gait, not to produce direct forward propulsion. For this reason these muscles need not be large and powerful. The extremities of the great runners in the animal kingdom are not well muscled. The relatively low mass of the extremity allows rapid flexion and extension without requiring tremendous energy to overcome the inertia of a large extremity. This is also true in the better human runners. During walking on a level surface the gastroc-soleus complex is active for approximately 20% to 50% of the stance phase of gait.[3] The calf muscles then cease activity before the roll-off stage of ambulation. The calf muscles are not used for push-off while walking or running. If we view the leg in relation to the foot, which is fixed on the ground, we see that the ankle undergoes dorsiflexion during the first half of the stance phase of gait. The angle between the tibia and the foot remains relatively unchanged for the second half of the stance phase of walking. Since the ankle is the major joint affected by the calf muscle, the gastroc-soleus complex undergoes first an eccentric contraction and then an isometric contraction. That is, it develops tension as it is being stretched for the first segment of the stance phase, and then it maintains the same length as the muscle further tenses (Fig. 10-1). This period corresponds to the heel being lifted off the floor. The calf muscle acts to stabilize the leg by restraining the forward motion of the tibia, therefore allowing the leg to act as a solid support for the body as it propels itself forward. During the isometric contraction the heel rises off the floor and the toes undergo passive dorsiflexion. Tension is then created dynamically in the plantar fascia, which assists in stabilizing the foot and the leg during the roll-off phase.

The action of the gastroc-soleus complex is somewhat different during running. The triceps surae of the runner becomes active at the end of the swing phase and continues to be active for the first 50% of the stance phase of gait. Initially the muscle undergoes an eccentric contraction to balance the sudden pull of the tibialis anterior muscle in preparation for heel strike. During the stance phase of gait the gastroc-soleus complex undergoes eccentric contraction to stabilize the lower extremity (Fig. 10-2). Instead of undergoing an isometric contraction, as in walking, the triceps surae complex ceases to be active and plantar flexion of the ankle begins. By mediating the rate of dorsiflexion of the ankle and flexion of the knee during the

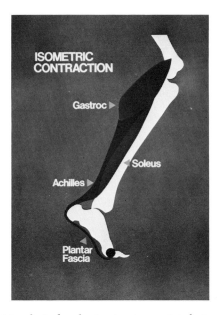

Fig. 10-1. Muscle is developing tension as it is being stretched.

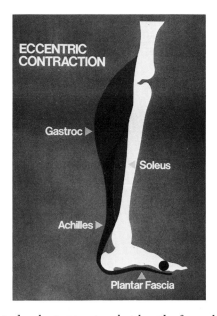

Fig. 10-2. Muscle is developing tension, but length of muscle remains constant.

stance phase of gait, the calf muscle also acts as an integral part of the shock-absorbing mechanism of the lower extremity. Because the calf muscle works mainly by an eccentric contraction, the muscle must be well stretched to allow its smooth elastic deformation during running. If the muscle is well stretched, tension develops more smoothly in the entire gastroc-soleus, Achilles tendon, and plantar fascia linkage system. A smooth elastic deformation of the muscle should take place without prematurely activating the stretch reflexes within the muscle and tendon unit, which would cause an abnormal, out-of-phase contraction.

EXAMINATION AND REHABILITATION

To rehabilitate a muscle group, the physician must determine if there is a problem within that muscle tendon unit. A careful history is important in determining

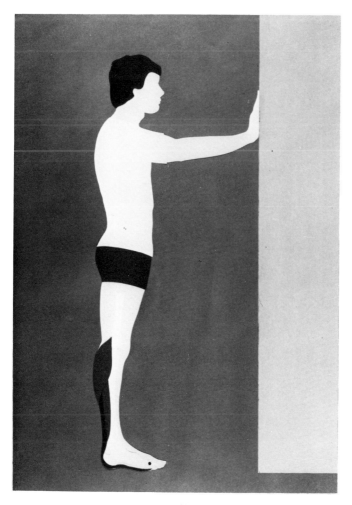

Fig. 10-3. Calf stretching.

if a pathological condition exists within the gastroc-soleus complex. Night cramps in the calf muscle or a cramping sensation in the toes after activity should alert the examiner to probable contracture in the complex. A history of pain under the plantar aspect of the heel or arch or in the triceps surae–Achilles tendon complex also suggests dynamic tightness of the calf. The physical examination should be conducted with the patient both standing and sitting. To determine contracture of the gastroc-soleus complex, the patient should hold the knee in extension and produce both passive and active dorsiflexion of the foot. If the foot can achieve dorsiflexion of 10 to 15 degrees beyond neutral, the muscle is said to be well stretched. If the foot cannot reach neutral dorsiflexion, there is a marked contracture of the gastrocnemius muscle. The same procedure should be followed with the knee flexed to determine a relative tightness in the soleus muscle. It should be noted that this is

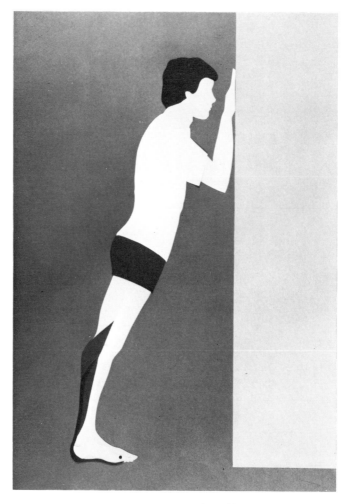

Fig. 10-4. Starting position for calf stretching.

a static test and therefore cannot show how well the muscle allows itself to be stretched during an eccentric contraction. Determining the dynamic stretchability of the gastroc-soleus complex is of key importance. Unfortunately, no test of this function has been developed. Therefore the history and associated physical findings must be used to determine the presence of dynamic tightness in the gastroc-soleus complex. It is rare to find weakness in this complex in a runner who does not have neurological problems.

Stretching exercises are important in the rehabilitation of the gastroc-soleus complex. These exercises should cause a plastic deformation in the muscle. Therefore the patient must do them when the muscles are relatively cool and not after a vigorous workout. When the muscles are warm and stretching is performed, an elastic deformation takes place. It is important to have the runner stretch at least three or four times a day before a workout. I use a program in which the patient stands at approximately arm's length from the wall with the feet together and kept flat on the floor (Fig. 10-3). The patient then bends the elbows and leans on the forearms with the back straight (Fig. 10-4). The patient stays in this position for 30 seconds and then comes back to a neutral position. This exercise should be done for four repetitions at least three or four times a day. Every few days the patient should attempt to move the feet a little farther from the wall. This routine can be modified slightly by working the tibialis anterior muscles with concentric or isometric contractions before doing the calf stretching. Some reports have shown that exercising the tibialis anterior muscles produces better plastic deformation of the calf muscles.

SUMMARY

The gastroc-soleus muscle complex, Achilles tendon, and plantar fascia should be viewed as a single linkage system. The main function of the gastroc-soleus complex is to restrain the forward motion of the tibia and therefore help stabilize the leg during the stance phase of gait. Also, by mediating the rate of flexion and extension of the ankle and knee, this complex aids in the shock-absorbing mechanism of the lower extremity. The gastroc-soleus complex must be well stretched to function properly.

REFERENCES

1. Hicks, J.H.: The mechanics of the foot. II. The plantar aponeurosis and the arch, Arch. J. Anat. **88:**25, 1954.
2. Inman, V.T.: The joints of the ankle, Baltimore, 1976, The Williams & Wilkins Co.
3. Mann, R.A., and Inman, V.T.: Phasic activity of the intrinsic muscles of the foot, J. Bone Joint Surg. **46A:**472, 1964.

11. Partial tears of the patellar tendon and the Achilles tendon

Rolf Ljungqvist
Ejnar Eriksson

Overuse syndromes involving various tendons have become common in the practice of sports medicine. This is due in part to the intensive training of top athletes, the poorly planned training programs for recreational athletes, and the increasing number of joggers. In runners the Achilles tendon is frequently affected and the patellar tendon is occasionally involved. Typical symptoms in these patients include burning and sometimes shooting or cutting pain after increased activity. Such cases are often mistakenly labeled tendinitis or peritendinitis. Ljunqvist in 1968[5] and 1977,[6] Blazina and co-workers in 1973,[1] and Clancy, Neidhart, and Brand in 1976[2] demonstrated that these patients often have partial ruptures or focal degeneration of their tendons. The aim of this chapter is to review briefly the diagnosis and treatment of partial rupture of the patellar and Achilles tendons.

PARTIAL PATELLAR TENDON TEAR

Although tendinitis or partial ruptures of the patellar tendon occur during running, they are more common in high jumping, basketball, and volleyball.[1,4,6,8] In a series of 80 patients undergoing surgery for this condition from 1968 to 1980, only 5% had sustained their injuries during running.

Diagnosis

The diagnosis of a partial rupture of the patellar tendon is based on the patient's history of pain during increased activity. Clinical investigation often reveals local swelling of the patellar tendon and distinct local tenderness on palpation. When palpating the tendon, the examiner can sometimes feel a defect. The diagnosis is also based on soft tissue x-ray studies of the tendon, which reveal local thickening obscuring the normal contrast between the tendon margin and the surrounding subcutaneous tissue. Ultrasonography reveals reduced echogenicity in the area of the partial tendon rupture (Fig. 11-1) and somewhat increased echogenicity in the surrounding granulation tissue.[9]

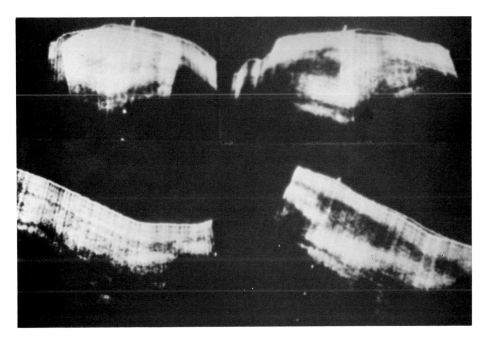

Fig. 11-1. Ultrasonography of patellar tendon with partial rupture *(upper and lower left)* and of normal tendon of other knee of same runner. In injured tendon, reduced echogenicity can be seen in both longitudinal and transverse sections. (Courtesy of L. Vedin, G. Westberg, and R. Ljungqvist, Seraphimerhospital, Stockholm, Sweden.)

Treatment

The treatment of patellar tendon rupture is surgical. Exposure is obtained in a bloodless field using a medial or lateral paraligamentous incision. The patellar tendon is carefully dissected through ventral and dorsal longitudinal incisions in the mesotenon. Near the apex of the patella, inflammatory adhesions between the tendon and the fat pad are often found. Rarely are ruptures observed in the tendon. However, when the tendon is carefully palpated, the surgeon can often feel a longitudinally oriented area of induration. If the tendon is carefully incised longitudinally over this region, yellow granulation tissue or even an empty space with hemorrhage and rounded ends of the partially ruptured fibers can be observed (Fig. 11-2). All granulation tissue and devitalized tendon is carefully excised. After this the tendon is closed side to side with absorbable synthetic suture material.

The postoperative treatment in the 80 cases reported consisted of a cylinder cast for 6 weeks followed by physical therapy and gradually increased training. A follow-up study of all the patients is now being performed and will be published later. In 1977 Ljungqvist published a report of his first nine cases, which he had followed for about 5 years. The results in these patients, who were high jumpers, were very good. The majority had improved function after surgery.

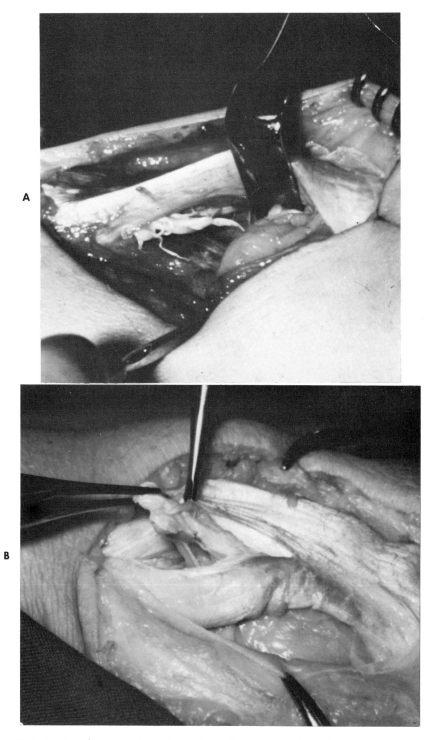

Fig. 11-2. A, Partial rupture in undersurface of patellar tendon. **B,** Old partial rupture of patellar tendon. Rupture could not be detected until tendon was incised longitudinally.

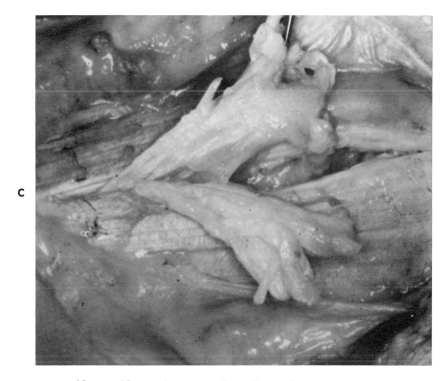

Fig. 11-2, cont'd. C, Old partial rupture of patellar tendon. Rupture ends became visible after tendon was incised longitudinally.

PARTIAL ACHILLES TENDON TEAR

Pain in the Achilles tendon is a very common complaint among runners and joggers. Many of these cases have erroneously been diagnosed as tendinitis or peritendinitis. During the period 1964 to 1980, 375 patients underwent surgery for this condition at the Seraphimerhospital in Stockholm.

Diagnosis

The diagnosis of a partial Achilles tendon rupture is based on the patient's complaint of shooting or cutting pain in the tendon, occurring after increased activity and often sudden in onset. The clinical examination commonly reveals an intensely painful area of thickening or induration that is irregular in contour. Reduced tonus in the gastrocnemius muscle and atrophy of the calf muscles are also found. If the rupture is of long duration, an increased passive dorsiflexion of the ankle joint exists. Soft tissue x-ray studies commonly show a pronounced thickening of the tendon. The contour of the tendon is often indistinct and not clearly distinguished from the subtendinous fat, and there seems to be a soft tissue infiltration into Kager's triangle. The soft tissue x-ray examination can be combined with ultrasonography and bursography.[9] Ultrasonography often reveals decreased echogenicity in the area of the partial rupture. Bursography of the subachilles bursa shows a path-

ological encroachment of the bursa into the Achilles tendon if there is a partial
rupture in the most distal portion of the tendon.

Electromyography (EMG) is often helpful in diagnosing a partial Achilles tendon
tear, as suggested by Persson and Ljungqvist.[7] EMG of both gastrocnemius bellies
is obtained with the patient resting and standing on his toes. In cases of partial
Achilles tendon rupture a reduction in the motor unit activity in the triceps surae
muscle connected to the area of partial rupture is found. If a rupture has occurred
in the soleus portion of the Achilles tendon, the time of contraction is shortened.
If the rupture has occurred in the gastrocnemius portion, the contraction time is

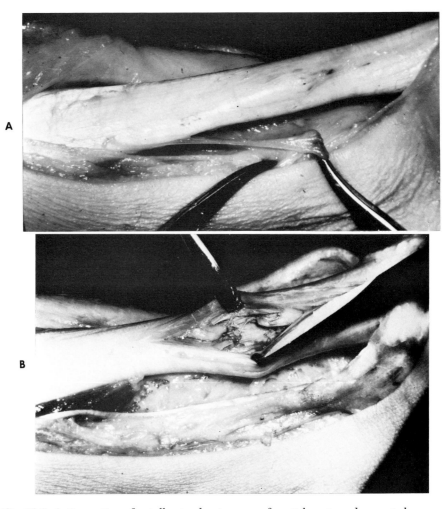

Fig. 11-3. A, Inspection of patellar tendon in cases of partial rupture does not always reveal
site of rupture. Thickening and discoloration, however, can be noted in one area. **B,** When
this area was incised, partial rupture was found. Adjacent tendon is also degenerated.

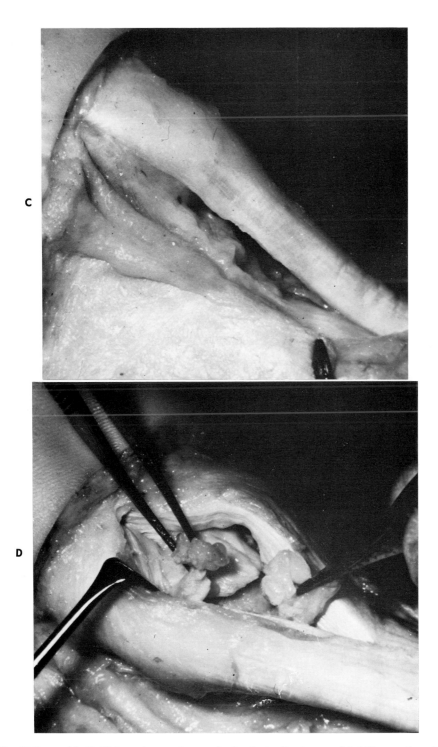

Fig. 11-3, cont'd. C, This patient, a jogger, had pain in distal part of Achilles tendon. Electromyographic investigation showed no abnormality, but bursography revealed contrast material leaking from deep bursa into tendon. This is usually a sign of partial rupture. **D,** Patient's tendon was incised longitudinally, revealing large partial rupture with ends that have been rounded off by attempts to heal.

prolonged and the contraction curve is deformed. An increased Hoffmann's reflex is found when the rupture has occurred in the soleus tendon portion. EMG, however, often shows no abnormality if the partial rupture has occurred close to the insertion of the Achilles tendon into the os calcis. Bursography commonly establishes the correct diagnosis in these cases.

Treatment

The treatment is surgery performed in a bloodless field. The peritenon is incised longitudinally, and the tendon is freed ventrally and dorsally. The findings within the tendon are exactly the same as described previously for the patellar tendon, but usually the area of involvement is more extensive (Fig. 11-3). The surgery consists of careful excision of all granulation tissue and devitalized tendon tissue. The tendon is sutured from side to side with synthetic absorbable suture material. If the partial tendon rupture is fairly large, a tendoplasty with the plantaris longus tendon can be performed. The plantaris longus tendon is tunneled into the defect and sutured to the distal end of the partial rupture. The postoperative treatment is a short leg cast for 3 weeks with the foot in moderate plantar flexion. This cast is then exchanged for a walking cast with the ankle in neutral flexion for another 3 weeks. The heel is elevated for the first few months of the patient's training. Normal physical therapy and a gradual return to training are recommended.

Results

Gillström and Ljungqvist[3] have recently published a 5-year follow-up report of the first 84 cases of partial Achilles tendon rupture treated at the Seraphimerhospital. Following surgery, 76% of the top athletes could return to competitive sports and 90% of the joggers could resume full physical activity. One patient established a world record for the 30-km run 1 year after surgery.

REFERENCES
1. Blazina, M.E., and others: Jumper's knee, Orthop. Clin. North Am. **4**:665, 1973.
2. Clancy, W.G., Neidhart, D., and Brand, R.L.: Achilles tendinitis in runners: a report of five cases, Am. J. Sports Med. **4**:45, 1976.
3. Gillström, P., and Ljungqvist, R.: Long-term results after operation for subcutaneous partial rupture of the Achilles tendon, Acta Chir. Scand. **482** (suppl.):78, 1978.
4. Johansson, S.: En förut icke beskriven sjukdom i patella, Hygiea **84**:161, 1922.
5. Ljungqvist, R.: Subcutaneous partial rupture of the Achilles tendon, Acta Orthop. Scand. **113** (suppl.):1, 1968.
6. Ljungqvist, R.: Partial subcutaneous ruptures of the patellar tendon. In Proceedings of the First Scandinavian Sportsmedicine Conference, 1977, Syntex Ter. **2**:89, 1977.
7. Persson, A., and Ljungqvist, R.: Electrophysiological observations in cases of partial and total ruptures of the Achilles tendon, Electroencephalogr. Clin. Neurophysiol. **31**:239, 1971.
8. Sinding-Larsen, M.: En hitil ukjendt sygdom i patellae, Norsk Magasin Laegevitenskap **82**:856, 1921.
9. Vedin, L., Westberg, G., and Ljungqvist, R.: Unpublished data.

12. Achilles tendon ruptures

Robert E. Leach

In 1967 and 1968 I read about six professional athletes whose careers were ended as the result of Achilles tendon ruptures. However, 3 years ago Nate Archibald, a guard in the National Basketball Association, tore his Achilles tendon and was operated on in Buffalo. Within 2 years he was able to return to the NBA with no apparent loss of his physical skills. None of these were track athletes, but the great running boom of the 1970s makes it inevitable that more Achilles tendon ruptures will occur in runners. Happily, there seems to be a significant change in the treatment philosophy since the 1960s so that today we can expect an athlete with an Achilles tendon rupture to be able to return to competition. This chapter discusses some aspects of the treatment and rehabilitation of athletes with Achilles tendon rupture.

I will not compare closed and open treatment of ruptures of the Achilles tendon in this discussion because I believe all Achilles tendon ruptures in athletes should be treated by surgical repair. I cannot imagine that any runner would want to take the chance of having decreased strength, power, and endurance in the posterior calf muscles, and it is my opinion based on reading and personal experience that closed treatment gives a poorer result than surgical repair.

An important study by Ingles and his associates[4] included 79 patients, 48 of whom were treated surgically and 31 nonsurgically. The patients treated nonsurgically attained only 72% of normal strength and 70% of normal power and endurance. The patients treated surgically were more satisfied with the results of their treatment. None of the surgically treated group had later ruptures of the Achilles tendon, whereas there were nine later ruptures in the group not treated surgically. There were two wound infections in the surgically treated patients, but both subsided without problems. The threat of infection or other surgical complications is not reason enough to consider the closed treatment of Achilles tendon ruptures in an athlete.

Achilles tendon ruptures tend to occur in athletic people, predominantly men in the third to fifth decades of life. As more women participate in sports, we will undoubtedly see more females in this group. Older runners will also be more susceptible to Achilles tendon ruptures, which we now see in the more mature tennis

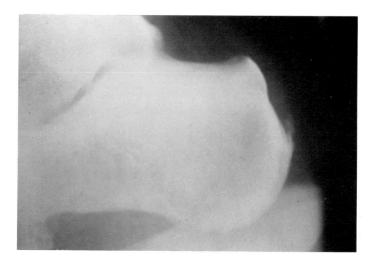

Fig. 12-1. Calcification within Achilles tendon.

and basketball players.[1,2] Most tendon ruptures occur 2 to 5 cm above the insertion into the os calcis in an area of the tendon that seems to have decreased vascularity.[5] The treating physician always wonders whether the rupture has occurred as the result of previous degeneration (Fig. 12-1) or a partial rupture of the tendon, as discussed by Dr. Eriksson, or whether it has occurred in a previously normal tendon solely as the result of greatly increased mechanical stress. From the patient's point of view the cause of the rupture is less important than that the diagnosis is made, treatment is adequate, and rehabilitation is supervised.

DIAGNOSIS

In most published series of ruptures of the Achilles tendon the diagnosis is missed in approximately 20% to 25% of the cases. This occurs partly because of the patient and partly because of the physician's error. Patients who have a rupture of the Achilles tendon do not have as much pain as they might expect from such a major tear. They hear a loud pop and have sudden pain that gradually subsides. Because of this subsidence of pain, they tend to minimize their complaints. In some instances they do not consult a physician immediately because they can walk, and they assume they could not if they had a major tear of the Achilles tendon. Blood accumulates in the tendon sheath, filling the defect in the tendon and making it difficult to detect (Fig. 12-2). When the plantaris tendon is intact, it and the plantar flexors of the toes allow some active plantar flexion of the foot, and the unwary physician may miss the defect. The patient is usually unable to stand on tiptoe on one foot, but he may tell the physician that this is because of pain. Thus the marked weakness of the posterior calf muscle group may be missed.

The test described by Thompson and Doherty[7] plays a vital part in the examination. It consists of squeezing the relaxed posterior calf muscles on the injured

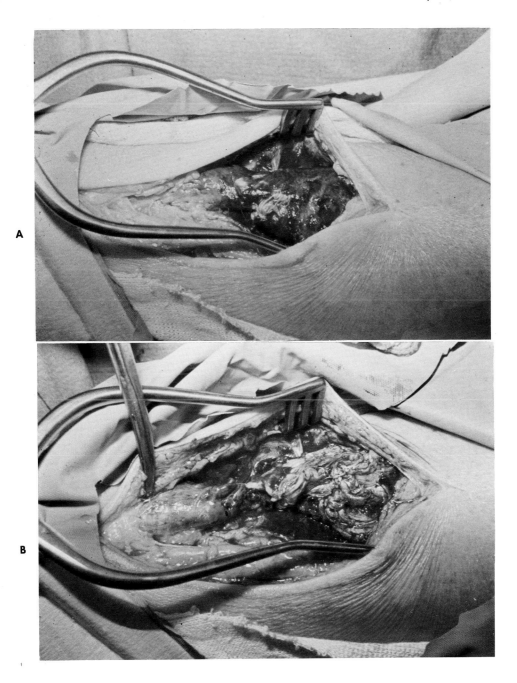

Fig. 12-2. A, Achilles rupture showing hematoma in intact sheath. **B,** Achilles rupture after incising sheath.

side. If plantar flexion of the foot occurs with that action, the Achilles tendon should be intact. If plantar flexion does not occur, the Achilles tendon is not intact. The careful examiner can usually palpate a defect in the Achilles tendon even though visual examination of the extremity does not suggest a ruptured tendon. There is a difference in palpable consistency between an entrapped hematoma and a normal intact tendon with its sheath.

OPERATIVE TREATMENT

Once the diagnosis of a ruptured Achilles tendon has been made, treatment should commence as soon as possible. As already stated, I would proceed with surgical repair. I have no experience with the percutaneous repair of the Achilles tendon described by Ma and Griffith[6] in 1977. The results of this treatment seem to be good, and it is an ingenious method of avoiding an open operation. However, the literature includes ample evidence that open surgery is also quite successful.

The surgeon must be careful (1) to avoid injuring the sural nerve, (2) to avoid damaging the overlying skin, and (3) to be sure the suture is strong and the tendon ends are held firmly together. There are a variety of ways of performing this procedure, among which are the use of percutaneous wire, the Bunnell stitch, and mattress stitches. I use a strong, synthetic suture with a figure of 8 as my primary holding stitch. In this way the tendon is sutured through both sides and both horizontally and vertically (Fig. 12-3). Following the holding stitch I use several other approximating sutures and close the tendon sheath. While placing the sutures, I keep the foot in plantar flexion and hold the fragmented tendon ends together. Although the tendon ends are often badly shredded, they will heal if sutured together. I try to restore the physiological tension and then reduce the plantar flexion toward neutral while watching the suture line to see where the foot is optimally held.

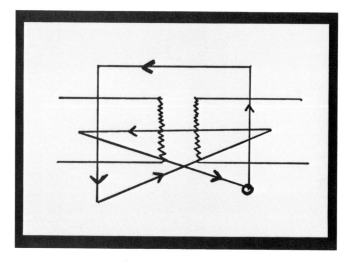

Fig. 12-3. Diagram of suture method for Achilles tendon repair.

POSTOPERATIVE CARE

The postoperative treatment is very important. Häggmark and Eriksson[3] have described hypotrophy of the soleus muscle after Achilles tendon rupture. Their thesis was that this muscle undergoes selective atrophy that is increased if tension is not kept on the tendon and the muscle. Therefore they recommended that the foot not be placed in plantar flexion but in as much dorsiflexion as possible while keeping the suture line intact. This is an important concept and is supported by other studies of immobilization of the ligaments and tendons. I put patients in a long leg cast with the knee slightly flexed to relieve stress on the gastrocnemius muscle and allow easier walking with crutches. The foot is placed in dorsiflexion to the level at which there appears to be no stress on the suture line. I have not had the courage to put stress on the suture line as Häggmark and Ericksson do. After 3 weeks I change the cast to a below-knee cast that allows the patient to straighten the leg and thus puts more tension on the suture line.

Six weeks after surgery I remove the cast and put the patient on crutches, asking him to wear a shoe with an elevated heel. He then begins weight-bearing on crutches until he can walk with a normal heel-toe gait. When that occurs, he begins to gradually lower the heel of the shoe and to perform stretching exercises of the posterior muscles of the calf. These are done by wall leaning and by placing

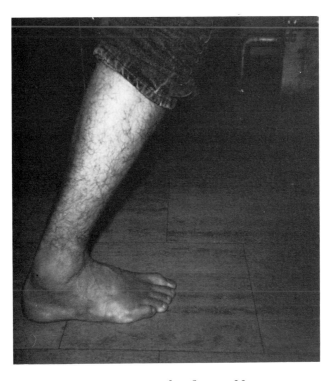

Fig. 12-4. Passive dorsiflexion of foot.

the affected foot forward with the heel flat on the ground and then bending the knee and the ankle, which produces stress on the posterior structures at the ankle (Fig. 12-4). Strengthening exercises begin with simple plantar flexion of the foot against no resistance and then against minor resistance provided by the hand of another person or by surgical tubing tied to a fixed point (Fig. 12-5). Gradually the patient progresses to toe stands, first on both legs with assistance, then on one leg with assistance, and finally on one leg without assistance. After some strength develops, the patient works with a machine that provides more resistance to active plantar flexion.

Some years ago I believed it would be almost impossible for a patient over 30 years of age who had an Achilles tendon rupture to develop normal calf strength and passive dorsiflexion. Now, however, I think that if a patient works hard, at the end of 6 to 7 months he can achieve nearly normal function. At the end of 1 year a number of these patients have test results in the normal range. To reach this point, however, they must work hard on both muscle strengthening and stretching. I also tell them to stretch diligently on the other side to prevent the other Achilles tendon from rupturing during activity.

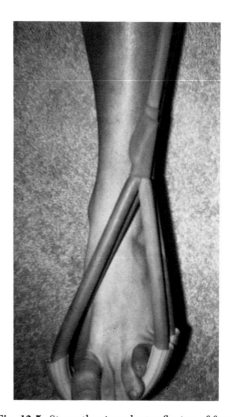

Fig. 12-5. Strengthening plantar flexion of foot.

One major problem in the treatment of Achilles tendon rupture occurs when the patient does not seek immediate treatment or when the diagnosis is delayed. If there is a gap in the tendon that has to be filled, the choices are few. I usually turn down a flap from the proximal portion of the tendon in the central area and use that as a graft to bridge the gap. The plantaris tendon can sometimes be used to bridge the gap, but it is usually too small and of little strength. Several patients with late surgical repair who worked hard afterward have been able to recover a muscle tendon complex with good strength and reasonable (but not usually normal) dorsiflexion.

I have not seen many track athletes who have sustained a complete rupture of the Achilles tendon, although partial ruptures are fairly common in this group. Several patients I operated on for this condition would probably have gone on to complete rupture if left untreated. A few of my track athlete patients have had complete ruptures. One was a steeplechase runner who made a bad misstep as he hit the edge of the board, causing acute dorsiflexion of his foot. Another hit the top of a wall as he was running cross country, resulting in dorsiflexion of his foot and tear of the Achilles tendon. As more people run for longer periods of time and particularly as more runners reach their thirties, forties, and fifties, Achilles tendon ruptures may become as common in track athletes as they now are in tennis and basketball players and skiers.

The most important aspect for a physician may be the treatment of chronic Achilles tendinitis and the partial ruptures that occur in this condition. If these are adequately treated and we can educate both the serious runners and the joggers to keep stretching and to pay attention to Achilles tendon symptoms, perhaps we will prevent Achilles tendon rupture in runners and leave it to the more violent sports.

REFERENCES

1. Clancy, W.G., Jr., Neidhart, D., and Brand, R.L.: Achilles tendinitis in runners: a report of five cases, Am. J. Sports Med. 4:76, 1976.
2. Denstad, T., and Roaas, A.: Surgical treatment of partial Achilles tendon ruptures, Am. J. Sports Med. 7:15, 1979.
3. Häggmark, T., and Eriksson, E.: Hypotrophy of the soleus muscle in man after Achilles tendon rupture: discussion of findings obtained by computed tomography and morphologic studies, Am. J. Sports Med. 7:121, 1979.
4. Ingles, A., and others: Ruptures of the tendo-Achilles: an objective assessment of the surgical and non-surgical treatment, J. Bone Joint Surg. 58A:990, 1976.
5. Lagengren, C., and Lindholm, A.: Vascular distribution in the Achilles tendon: an angiographic and microangiographic study, Acta Chir. Scand. 116:491, 1958-1959.
6. Ma, G.W.C., and Griffith, T.G.: Percutaneous repair of acute closed ruptures of Achilles tendon: a new technique, Clin. Orthop. Rel. Res. 128:247, 1977.
7. Thompson, T.C., and Doherty, J.H.: Spontaneous rupture of tendon of Achilles: a new diagnostic clinical test, J. Trauma 2:126, 1962.

13. Knee pain in the middle-aged runner

Ejnar Eriksson
Tom Häggmark

With the growing interest in jogging, a number of runners over the age of 40 years with early signs of degenerative arthritis of the knee joints complain of pain and a tendency to effusion of one or both knee joints after running.

It is normally useless to tell these enthusiastic joggers to give up jogging, but the physician can sometimes persuade them to reduce their mileage. Some of them, however, continue to have symptoms and request treatment. In such cases we use a therapy suggested in 1934 by Burman, Finkelstein, and Mayer.[1] They reported that some of their arthritic patients were symptom free for long periods after arthroscopy and washing out of their knee joints. Chrisman, Fessel, and Southwick[2] have given a possible explanation as to why washing out the knee joints might be helpful for patients with mild arthritis. They produced symptomatic synovitis in dogs by injecting small fragments of the cartilage of one knee joint into the other knee joint. It is therefore possible that small fragments of joint cartilage worn off the joint during extensive running can cause synovitis. It is reasonable to believe that if these small pieces of cartilage are washed out, the symptoms of synovitis may diminish.

Table 13-1. Knee lavage treatment of arthritis in joggers

Patient no.	Sex	Age	Arthritis*	Years of treatment	Interval between treatments (months)
1	Male	55	+	2	8
2	Male	60	+	3	6
3	Male	62	+ +	2	6
4	Male	52	+	3	12
5	Male	57	+ +	2	6
6	Female	41	+ +	3	4
7	Male	53	+	4	6
8	Male	65	+ +	2	8
9	Male	58	+	2	8
10	Male	55	+	3	6

*+, Mild; + +, moderate.

106

MATERIAL AND METHODS

A group of 10 joggers, 41 to 65 years of age (Table 13-1), was examined with arthroscopy for complaints of pain and swelling of one or both knees after jogging. Arthroscopic examination of all the knees revealed arthritis of varying degree. All improved after arthroscopy. These patients have been treated with regular lavage of the joint at varying intervals of 4 to 12 months. The subsequent joint irrigations were performed with a syringe and a large-bore needle and not by arthroscopy.

RESULTS

All 10 runners have been able to continue running during a period of observation of 2 to 4 years with a new lavage of the knee joint every 4 to 12 months (Table 13-1). The following are the case histories of two typical patients in this group.

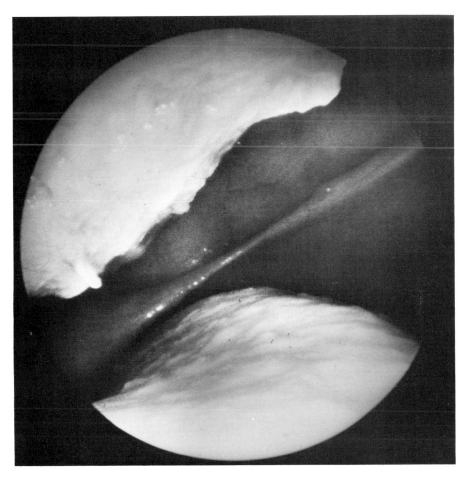

Fig. 13-1. Gas arthroscopy of knee joint of 52-year-old man with mild to moderate signs of arthritis who has been treated with repeated knee lavages. (From Eriksson, E., and Sebik, A.: Orthop. Clin. North Am. **13**:293, 1982.)

CASE 4

This patient is a 52-year-old musician who has participated in jogging for the last 4 to 5 years. He first consulted us in 1976 for an acutely swollen knee. X-ray examination revealed mild signs of arthritis. Gas arthroscopy showed the degree of arthritis and chondromalacia (Fig. 13-1). During the arthroscopy the knee was carefully washed out and subsequently improved so much that 3 weeks later he could resume jogging. When symptoms returned after about 12 months, he returned for a second knee lavage. This made him symptom free for another 12 months. He usually jogs 3 to 4 miles two or three times a week without any problems. He was recently treated for a similar problem in his other knee where the same degree of arthritis was found. After an arthroscopic knee lavage the second knee has been symptom free for over a year.

CASE 8

A 65-year-old physician showed moderate signs of arthritis on x-ray examination. He had been physically active all his life and sought treatment 2 years ago because of pain and effusion in his right knee joint after jogging. Arthroscopy revealed no explanation for his pain and joint effusion other than a moderate degree of arthritis. The knee was carefully washed out, and he resumed jogging 3 to 4 weeks after the arthroscopy. He has subsequently returned three times at 8-month intervals for knee lavage. He says that he is completely symptom free since the knee lavage procedures and is able to jog 4 miles three or four times a week.

DISCUSSION

If a patient over 40 years of age complains of swelling and knee pain resulting from jogging, the knee should be carefully examined to rule out a meniscus disorder, ligamentous injuries, or other nonarthritic conditions. Arthroscopy combined with a careful clinical investigation has a high degree of accuracy. If arthroscopy shows no reason for the knee pain other than mild to moderate arthritis with synovitis and the runner does not want to give up running or reduce his mileage considerably (which should be the first recommendation), knee lavage can alleviate the symptoms. We believe that among the many different types of treatment available, such as nonsteroidal anti-inflammatory agents, long-term salicylate treatment, and local corticosteroid injections, knee lavage is probably the least dangerous. Furthermore, it has to be repeated only occasionally. Therefore we advocate this treatment in selected cases of very highly motivated runners who wish to continue running in spite of mild to moderate arthritis of the knee joint.

REFERENCES

1. Burman, M.S., Finkelstein, H., and Mayer, L.: Arthroscopy of the knee joint, J. Bone Joint Surg. 16A:255, 1934.
2. Chrisman, O.D., Fessel, J.M., and Southwick, W.O.: Experimental production of synovitis and marginal articular exostosis in the knee joints of dogs, Yale J. Biol. Med. 37:409, 1965.

14. Stress fractures in runners, excluding the foot

Douglas W. Jackson
Alan M. Strizak

A stress or fatigue fracture occurs when the bone's ability to accommodate to the repetitive demands placed on it is exceeded. A stress fracture differs from an acute fracture in that it is a summation of repeated subclinical stresses over a period of time rather than a single traumatic event. Bone is a living tissue. It is in a constant state of turnover, adjusting as needed to stresses imposed on it. Manifestations of a breakdown in the bone's ability to accommodate and remodel may vary from a radiographic reaction to intramedullary changes to partial or complete breaks in the continuity of the cortices of the bone. Stress fractures are easily diagnosed when they are radiographically apparent. Subradiographic (microscopic) stress fractures are more common than was once thought and are less easily recognized. Bone pain that progressively increases during running should raise the question of a subradiographic stress fracture. The majority of stress reactions in runners heal without a diagnosis ever being made.

Stress fractures have been described as resembling fatigue fractures in metal.[1,13,14,22] Experiments using isolated bone fragments under cyclic loading[4,18,23] have failed to take into account the effects of the muscle mass that surrounds bone in vivo and can either decrease or increase the variables in the stress applied. The role of fatigue of the supporting musculature with the resultant increased stress transmitted directly to the bone has been incriminated in stress fractures in runners. It is unclear to what degree this mechanism is important in the genesis of fatigue fractures. In some fatigue fractures direct weight-bearing plays no part in the cause. Examples of this are rib fractures resulting from chronic cough and fractures of the upper extremities seen in tennis players and baseball players.

Stress fractures in runners appear to result when repetitive pounding and muscular action on the lower extremity exceed the strength and reparative capacity of the bone.[19] Stress fractures have been demonstrated in only two species other than humans, both of which are involved in running under the supervision of humans: the race horse[10] and the racing greyhound.[7]

Stress fractures represent an entire spectrum of breakdown in the bone's ability to accommodate to the demands of the runner.[9] The majority of these problems are limited to subradiographic changes confirmed only by a technetium pyrophosphate bone scan or by serial x-ray studies that eventually show intramedullary changes, disruption of one cortex, or merely focal cortical hypertrophy. The important factors determining whether the runner develops a stress fracture are the stress imposed and the time period over which it occurs.

In addition, certain runners seem more susceptible to stress fractures. These individuals often have more than one stress fracture during their running careers and have stress fractures at a lower mileage. The majority of runners, however, do not allow more than one stress fracture to occur. They pay attention to training pains and do not try to "run through" their bone pain. Stress fractures are usually related to an error in training and occur after the runner (1) changes surfaces, (2) changes shoes, (3) includes hill work, (4) changes the intensity of interval work, or (5) increases mileage.

In vitro bovine bone exposed to flexural fatigue develops macroscopic fracture patterns similar to those resulting from a single bending load. Microscopically, however, progressive accumulation of diffuse structural damage can be demonstrated in the flexural fatigue specimen before complete failure. Carter and Hayes[5] concluded that the diffuse nature of the observed fatigue damage is consistent with the hypothesis that microdamage caused by mechanical loading may serve as a stimulus for in vivo bone remodeling.

Radiographic documentation of stress fractures was described by Stechow[20] in 1897. This evidence is of course delayed until adequate time has occurred for resorption of local bone and/or formation of new bone that can be detected radiographically. Thus x-ray studies are less sensitive and less useful in the evaluation of early and less advanced stress fractures. The recent advent of the technetium pyrophosphate bone scan has made it possible to identify lesions that develop and heal at subradiographic levels (Fig. 14-1). The scan can detect lesions within 3 to 5 days of the onset of the patient's bone pain. The use of the bone scan in competitive runners permits early treatment and minimizes recovery time. This is of particular importance to athletes involved in high levels of intense training, since a prolonged period of unnecessary inactivity would seriously set them back.

Fig. 14-2 shows a biopsy specimen from an area of increased uptake on a radioactive isotope study in a young athlete whose x-ray studies showed no abnormalities. The fractured bone spicule demonstrates callus formation. This microfracture of a spicule of bone was among intact spicules. The fracture healed without being detectable on follow-up x-ray examination. The accumulation of this type of microtrauma eventually results in the radiographic changes that have been typically described as stress fractures.

The radiographic evaluation of an early stress fracture is usually negative at the onset of bone pain, and commonly as long as 2 to 3 weeks is required to appreciate an abnormality in the bone. The diagnosis is based on a careful examination and

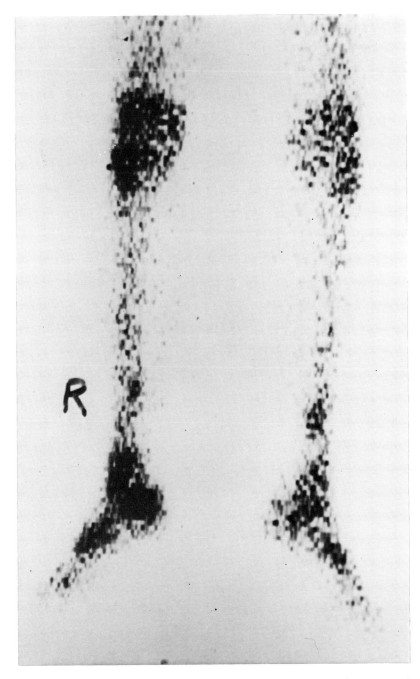

Fig. 14-1. Bilateral increased uptake in this technetium pyrophosphate bone scan of runner correlated with localized bone pain.

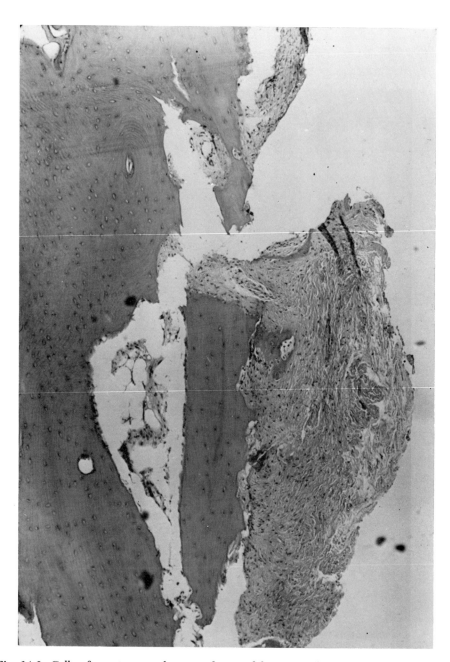

Fig. 14-2. Callus formation in relation to fractured bony spicule represents microfracture. This bone biopsy of proximal tibia was obtained in young athlete with no radiologic abnormalities and a positive bone scan.

localization of the pain and tenderness to the bone. The adjacent soft tissue is often swollen, which may confuse those unfamiliar with the early manifestations of a stress fracture. The radioisotope bone scan is unnecessary for diagnosis if one is aware of the early findings in a runner. The changes in uptake on the bone scan usually subside within 1 to 3 months but may remain for 1 to 2 years in athletes who continue to run despite their symptoms.

DIFFERENTIAL DIAGNOSIS

The differential diagnosis of stress fractures in runners includes osteoid osteoma, osteomyelitis, osteogenic sarcoma, Paget's disease, and other infectious processes

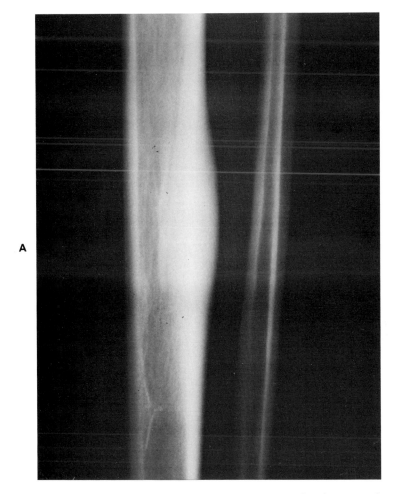

A

Fig. 14-3. A, Cortical hypertrophy in young runner was considered a stress fracture. The possibility of osteoid osteoma was entertained. Nidus could not be demonstrated on routine x-ray examination, but computed tomography revealed nidus and confirmed diagnosis of osteoid osteoma.   *Continued.*

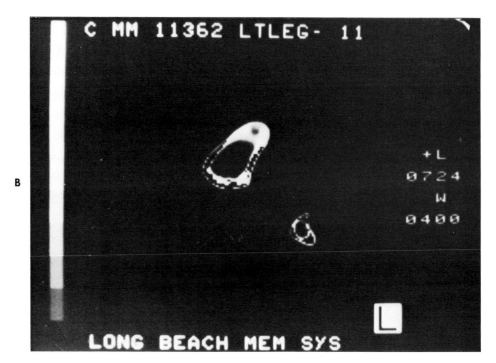

Fig. 14-3, cont'd. B, Nidus as seen on computed tomogram.

and tumors that result in periosteal reactions or peripheral bony destruction. An osteoid osteoma may rarely be a confusing problem in the younger patient who complains of bone pain and local tenderness in association with running. The following factors are helpful in the differential diagnosis: (1) stress fractures tend to occur at typical locations; (2) serial x-ray studies change more rapidly in cases of stress fracture; (3) stress fractures are usually associated with pain during running, which is relieved by non-weight-bearing; (4) it is unusual for a stress fracture to be associated with pain at night; (5) osteoid osteomas seem to respond more dramatically to aspirin than do stress fractures; and (6) the pain associated with a stress fracture tends to be focal rather than scleratomal.

Computed tomography has been useful in evaluating cortical lesions when it is not clear whether a stress fracture is developing. Fig. 14-3 illustrates a dramatic osteoid osteoma that had been confused with a cortical stress fracture in a young distance runner.

SPECIFIC STRESS FRACTURE SITES
Lumbar spine

Spondylolysis developing as an acute stress fracture in a runner is unusual.[16] However, this fracture may develop in young runners who are participating in another sport requiring lumbar hyperextension and jarring activities. The running aggravates the developing bony reaction in the pars interarticularis. Stress fractures in the pars interarticularis are atypical in terms of those seen elsewhere in the body:

1. There is often a family predisposition in the development of an acute pars interarticularis stress fracture.
2. There is a higher incidence of dysplasia in the posterior elements of the lumbar spine.
3. The fracture commonly results in a nonunion (this is very unusual in stress fractures).

Because of the difficulty of obtaining adequate radiographic evaluation of the pars interarticularis, the technetium bone scan has been helpful in delineating acute (recent) stress reactions in this area. Fig. 14-1 depicts a pars interarticularis defect that is well established. These established defects are an incidental finding in the lumbar spines of many runners.

Pelvis

Stress fractures of the pubic rami and the pubic bone, accompanied by pubic symphysitis, occur infrequently but can be refractory to treatment.[17] When unexplained pain occurs in the area of the symphysis pubis or pubic rami, a technetium pyrophosphate bone scan may show increased activity. Stress reaction and inflammation of the pubis symphysis tend to occur in distance runners who are also doing abdominal-strengthening exercises. The pubic reaction may be associated with strenuous use of the rectus abdominis and adductor muscles. These runners can usually bicycle without pain but have increasing pain when attempting to run.

It often takes 3 to 6 months and may take up to 1 year of restriction from running to eliminate a refractory stress reaction and inflammation of the symphysis pubis. A local corticosteroid injection can provide transient relief for 2 to 4 weeks and may allow the runner to participate in an important competition before undertaking a period of rest. In addition to aiding the evaluation of the pubis and symphysis pubis, the bone scan gives some indication of sacroiliac joint involvement. A specific history should be taken to determine the presence of underlying urological symptoms including urethral discharges, involvement of other joints with arthralgias, rashes, and changes in the mucous membranes and eyes.

Hip

The femoral neck is one of the few stress fracture sites in which operative intervention may be indicated.[2] Stress fractures in the hip are more common in military recruits than in the general running population. Femoral neck fractures often begin with changes in the inferior cortices of the femoral neck. If detected early enough, they can be treated with crutches and non-weight-bearing, but percutaneous pinning allows earlier weight-bearing without concern for displacement of the fracture.

Stress fractures of the lesser trochanter are unusual. They should be suspected in patients with discomfort at the insertion of the hip flexors. These stress fractures may be differentiated from bursitis and tendinitis by positive findings on a bone scan or changes on serial x-ray studies.

Femoral shaft

The medial one third of the shaft of the femur is an infrequent site of stress fractures in distance runners, and displacement of stress fractures of the femoral shaft is uncommon in the civilian running population. However, these fractures have occurred in top-level athletes, as Fig. 14-4 shows. The pain pattern may be confusing, and a stress fracture should be suspected in runners with pain in the thigh that cannot be well localized. If detected early, these fractures respond to rest and restricted motion. Significant cortical hypertrophy may occur during the healing process.

Patella

The patella may be the site of a stress fracture, although this is unusual. The stress fracture may be vertical or transverse, and the history is that of gradually

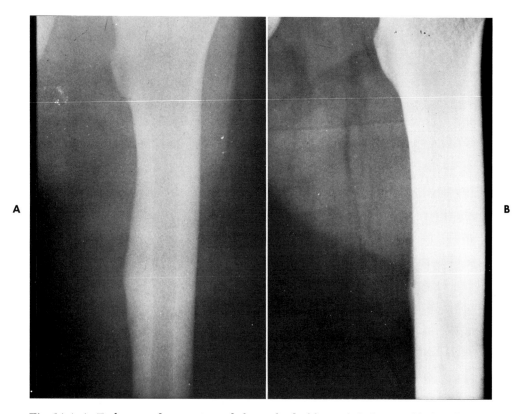

Fig. 14-4. A, Early stress fracture in medial one third of femoral shaft in world-class distance runner. This stress reaction developed 6 weeks before Olympic trials. **B,** Follow-up x-ray study shows cortical hypertrophy associated with healing.

increasing pain during vigorous activity without significant injury. Stress fracture of the patella may be confused with chondromalacia. Special x-ray views and a bone scan may be necessary to demonstrate the fracture. Displacement of a patellar fracture may require surgical internal fixation.

Tibia

The tibia is the most common site of stress fractures in distance runners.[3,6,15] This varies to some degree among running populations. In runners who run more than 20 miles a week, the thick cortical bone of the tibia tends to become vulnerable to stress fractures. The most common bony reaction in runners occurs along the posteromedial aspect of the tibia approximately 12 to 13 cm proximal to the tip of the medial malleolus (Fig. 14-5). This area is just distal to the muscle attachment

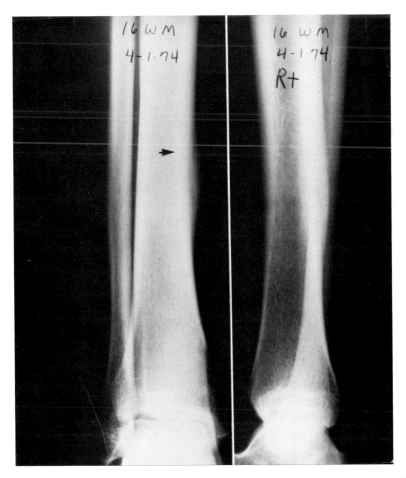

Fig. 14-5. Posterior medial tibial discomfort developed approximately 12 cm proximal to tip of medial malleolus in young runner, who continued running in spite of pain and went on to develop full-blown stress fracture shown here. Arrow indicates x-ray change.

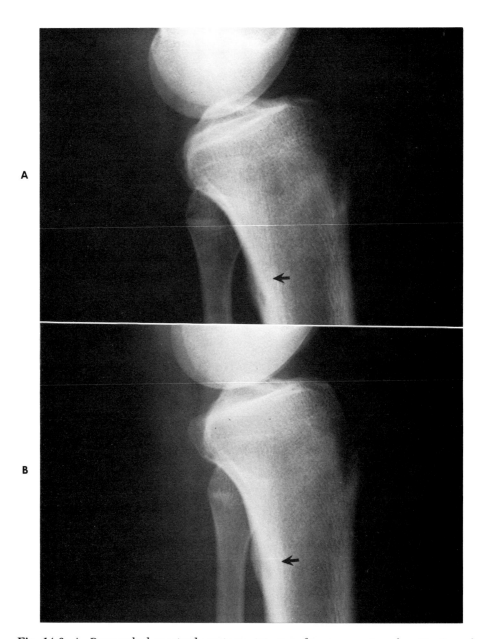

Fig. 14-6. A, Runner had received cortisone injection for pes anserinus bursitis 6 weeks before this x-ray study. **B,** Three months later, bony defect showed radiologic evidence of healing. Runner resumed training without tibial pain. Arrows in **A** and **B** indicate x-ray changes.

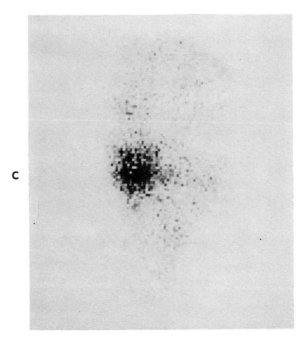

Fig. 14-6, cont'd. C, Increased uptake on technetium pyrophosphate scan is confined to medial tibial plateau. This correlated with runner's bony tenderness and pain.

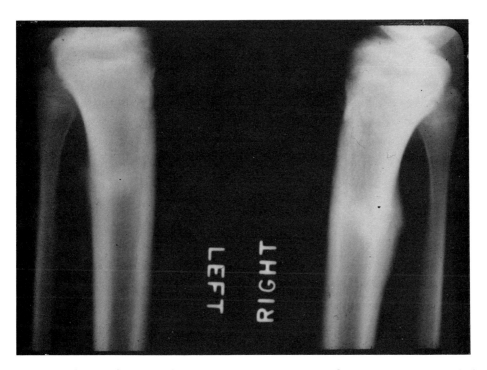

Fig. 14-7. Bilateral tibial stress fractures in young cross-country distance runner. Patient had had two corticosteroid injections into area of discomfort before development of x-ray changes.

on the posteromedial aspect of the tibia, and it is an area where cortical hypertrophy occurs in many younger runners. This can be associated with shin pain and is detected by a bone scan. More advanced cases of cortical disruption and periosteal reaction are detectable with x-ray studies. Stress reactions and fractures in this area may also be confused with posterior tibial tendinitis, periosteal reaction, or deep posterior compartment syndrome. Bony ridges may be palpated along the cortices with the new periosteal bone buildup. The localized tenderness is not aggravated by motion of the tendons and can be detected by direct palpation. Usually the clinical diagnosis is enough to confirm a bony reaction, although special x-ray studies or a bone scan may be required. Athletes undergoing vigorous training should take steps to prevent the development of stress fractures in the tibia and should respect the early warning pain.

The proximal tibia along the posteromedial plateau may also be the site of a stress fracture, which is commonly confused with pes anserinus bursitis (Fig. 14-6).[12] The bone pain may be associated with intermedullary changes and eventual cortical disruption.

The third area commonly involved with a tibial stress fracture is just distal to

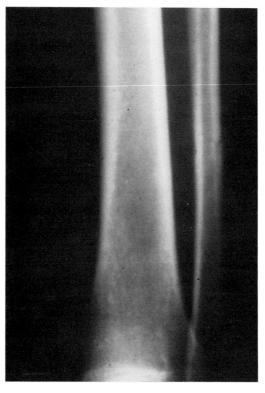

Fig. 14-8. Early stress fracture of fibula was present on x-ray films taken 4 weeks after onset of symptoms.

the tibial tubercle. Stress fractures in this site commonly occur in young runners and may be associated with a marked periosteal reaction (Fig. 14-7).[8] These stress fractures have occasionally been confused with a malignancy by those not familiar with this problem. Bony tenderness associated with increased periosteal activity is usually the basis for the diagnosis.

Fibula

Stress fractures of the fibula tend to occur in inexperienced runners. They usually occur in the distal one half of the fibula and are easily diagnosed because of the ease of palpation of the fibula and the presence of localized bony tenderness. It may take 2 to 4 weeks for x-ray studies to show evidence of the fracture, but close scrutiny of the x-ray films with a magnifying lens and bright light often reveals the early disruption of the fibular cortices (Fig. 14-8).[11] More proximal stress fractures of the fibula have been reported in military recruits.[21] These were attributed to vigorous jumping exercises from a full squatting position several times a day.

SUMMARY

Bone pain occurring in runners as they increase mileage or the intensity of their interval work is often associated with a breakdown in the remodeling process of the bone. If the bone does not have time to adapt to the new stress applied to it, it may fatigue and the microscopic trauma may proceed to a macroscopic level detectable on x-ray examination. Because this potential exists in all runners, running programs should include adequate stretching, muscle strengthening, and graduated loading of the bones. Increases in training intensity and mileage should be reasonable, and time should be allowed for adjusting to new shoes, different running surfaces, and hills. Running with leg pain may result in the establishment of more advanced stress fractures and may cause the runner to miss a significant part of a running season. Stress fractures have had an increased incidence in young women, particularly those in organized running events in high school who begin the cross-country season without adequate preseasoning and a year-round maintenance program. However, the discrepancy in incidence between men and women is decreasing as more women participate in year-round running programs and their bones become conditioned to the new demands.

Stress fractures respond to rest, and less advanced stress reactions may respond to an orthotic device. On occasion, however, a cast may be necessary for immobilization while the reparative process takes place. Once a stress fracture becomes apparent, usually 6 weeks to 3 months is required before the runner can resume a running program. The runner should return to a graduated program, paying attention to bone pain and giving the bone time to adjust to the new stresses.

REFERENCES

1. Baker, J., Frankel, V.H., and Burstein, A.H.: Fatigue fractures: biomechanical considerations, J. Bone Joint Surg. **54A**:1345, 1972.
2. Blickenstaff, L.D., and Morris, J.M.: Fatigue fracture of the femoral neck, J. Bone Joint Surg. **48A**:1031, 1966.

3. Burrows, H.J.: Fatigue infraction of the middle of the tibia in ballet dancers, J. Bone Joint Surg. **38B**:83, 1956.
4. Burstein, A.H., and Frankel, V.H.: A standard test for laboratory animal bone, J. Biomech. **4**:155, 1971.
5. Carter, D.R., and Hayes, W.C.: Compact bone fatigue damage, Clin. Orthop. **127**:265, 1977.
6. Devas, M.B.: Longitudinal stress fractures, J. Bone Joint Surg. **42B**:508, 1960.
7. Devas, M.B.: Compression stress fractures in man and the greyhound, J. Bone Joint Surg. **43B**:540, 1961.
8. Devas, M.B.: Stress fractures in children, J. Bone Joint Surg. **45B**:528, 1963.
9. Devas, M.B.: Stress fractures, London, 1975, Churchill Livingstone.
10. Devas, M.B.: Stress fractures, New York, 1975, Longman Publishing Co.
11. Devas, M.B., and Sweetnam, R.: Stress fracture of the fibula, J. Bone Joint Surg. **38B**:818, 1956.
12. Engber, W.D.: Stress fractures of the medial tibial plateau, J. Bone Joint Surg. **59A**:767, 1977.
13. Evans, F.G.: Stress and strain in bones, Springfield, Ill., 1957, Charles C Thomas, Publishers.
14. Hartley, J.B.: "Stress" or fatigue fractures of bone, Br. J. Radiol. **16**:255, 1943.
15. Jackson, D.W.: Shinsplints: an update, Phys. Sportsmed. **6**:51, 1978.
16. Jackson, D.W., and others: Stress fractures of the pars interarticularis in young athletes, Am J. Sports Med. **9**:305, 1981.
17. Koch, R., and Jackson, D.W.: Pubic symphysitis in distance runners, Am. J. Sports Med. **9**:62, 1981.
18. Puhl, J.J., Piotrowski, G., and Enneking, W.F.: Biomechanical properties of paired canine fibulas, J. Biomech. **5**:391, 1972.
19. Stanitski, C.L., McMaster, J.H., and Scranton, P.E.: On the nature of stress fractures, Am. J. Sports Med. **6**:391, 1978.
20. Stechow, A.W.: Fussoedem und roentgenstrahlen, Dtsch. Mil.-Aerztl. Zeitg. **26**:465, 1897.
21. Symeonides, P.P.: High stress fractures of the fibula, J. Bone Joint Surg. **42B**:508, 1960.
22. Trueta, J.: Studies of the development and decay of the human frame, Philadelphia, 1968, W.B. Saunders Co.
23. Yamada, H.: Strength of biological materials, edited by F. Gaynor Evans, Baltimore, 1970, The Williams & Wilkins Co.

15. Low back problems in runners

Douglas W. Jackson
Allan N. Sutker

Lumbar spine pain and disability may result from running or may develop in an unrelated activity and be accentuated and prolonged by running. The increasing number of runners participating in regular distance training, including marathons, has resulted in larger numbers with localized or referred pain in the lumbar spine. As in the general population, runners most commonly experience their back restrictions between the ages of 30 and 60 years.

Low back pain is something that most adults experience at some time during their lifetime. Man's unique upright posture and the repetitive demands placed on the lumbar spine may be contributing factors.[5] The runner in particular places repetitive demands of hyperextension and cyclic loading on the lumbar spine, aggravating and prolonging what otherwise would be mild symptoms. However, in a prospective study of 1077 adult runners seeking treatment for disabling musculoskeletal complaints, only 11 had disability related to the lumbar spine.[9]

The incidence of spinal complaints varies depending on the sampling of the runner population. The average age of the runners being evaluated is important because spinal complaints are uncommon in runners under the age of 25. Determining the exact incidence of spinal problems in the running population is further complicated because the majority of spinal symptoms are of an aching nature and only intermittently are severe enough to restrict the runner's mileage. Athletes are active people who often accept their spinal discomfort without seeking formal medical advice.

EXAMINATION OF THE RUNNER

Runners with lumbar spine disability require the same detailed examination as nonrunners. Runners, however, usually want a specific explanation for their pain, and they want a recommendation and a prognosis that do not curtail their running. Specific questions to runners provide helpful information to the physician. Of particular interest are the severity of pain in relation to running, the type of running program, the terrain, the surface, the time of day, the shoe type and style, the miles per week, the time the patient has been running, and the farthest the patient has run at one time.

In addition to the history, a pictorial representation of the runner's pain is help-ful in deciding whether the pain is localized or referred (Fig. 15-1).[10,11] The pres-ence of an associated dermatomal or sclerotomal distribution is important in assess-ing spinal pain. Runners with referred pain, particularly radicular pain, require more complete restriction than those with localized lumbar discomfort.

More attention should be paid to leg length discrepancies in distance runners than in the general population. These can be evaluated by many different methods. Measurements from the anterosuperior iliac crest to the medial malleoli do not provide information concerning the foot structure. An x-ray film of the pelvis made with the patient standing takes into account the entire lower extremity, including the weight-bearing structure. For example, when one foot is more pronated than the other, it contributes to a relative leg length discrepancy during weight-bearing. We have treated runners with low back discomfort who had a discrepancy of greater than 1 cm in leg length. The question of which leg length discrepancies are con-tributing factors is a multivariable one. A lift is an innocuous treatment and can be tried empirically, since it is inexpensive and seldom aggravates the underlying problem.

The radiographic evaluation of the lumbar spine in the runner complaining of pain is usually of little help in diagnosis, management, or prognosis. We obtained lumbar spine x-ray studies of 71 asymptomatic marathon runners.[16] The incidence of degenerative changes was close to that in the general population of similar age (Fig. 15-2). The incidence of degenerative changes corresponded most directly to the runner's age and not to the years of running or mileage run.[15] However, in a study of another group of athletes (weightlifters), Aggrawal and co-workers[1] found a higher incidence of spondyloloses (osteophyte formations) and Schmorl's nodes than in the general population.

Even significant lumbosacral spine x-ray changes are not directly correlated with the magnitude of symptoms.[13] The presence of radiographic changes in the lumbar spine does not preclude the runner from running unlimited mileage. These changes may or may not be associated with a particular pain complex. Runners with mild radiographic changes do not seem to have greater spine problems than those with-out changes.

Supplemental diagnostic tests beyond the routine lumbar x-ray survey of the spine in the runner are seldom necessary. Electromyography, myelography, spinal fluid analysis, venography, bone scan, computed tomography, segmental nerve blocks, thiopental examinations, and psychometric evaluations are part of the ar-mamentarium for those with negative results of x-ray examination. In the differen-tial diagnosis the physician must consider not only mechanical discogenic repetitive microtrauma, tendinitis, fasciitis, and stress fractures but also infections and neo-plastic processes.

The distance runner as a rule does not have secondary gains and psychological problems that interfere with recovery, as is often the case with patients being treated for spinal complaints who have lawsuits and industrial compensation judg-

Be sure to fill this out extremely accurately. Mark the area on your body
where you feel the described sensation. Use the appropriate symbol. Mark
areas of radiation. Include all affected areas.

Numbness ▰▰▰   Pins and needles ▨▨   Burning pain ×××××   Stabbing pain ////   Aching pain ((((

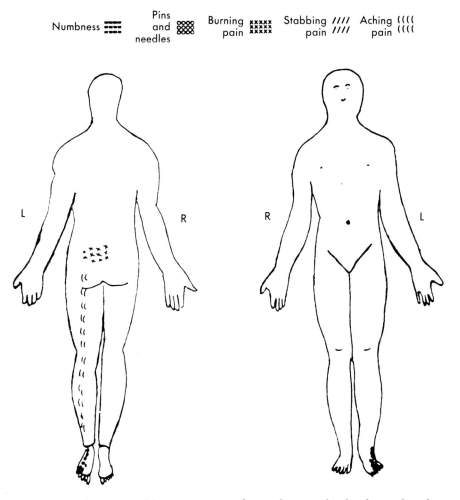

Fig. 15-1. Pain drawing used by runners to indicate if pain is localized or referred in its distribution.

ments pending. However, the psychological aspects of not being able to run present a specific problem in the runner. The physician seldom has to recommend on the initial visit that the runner give up running to solve his spinal complaints. However, restricted mileage or complete rest may be part of the initial treatment. The majority of runners eventually return to unrestricted running, and reassurance of this during the first visit provides emotional relief to the runner.

Runners with intermittent referred pain or minimal or subtle physical findings often pose difficulties in diagnosis. It is not uncommon to have a nonspecific pain

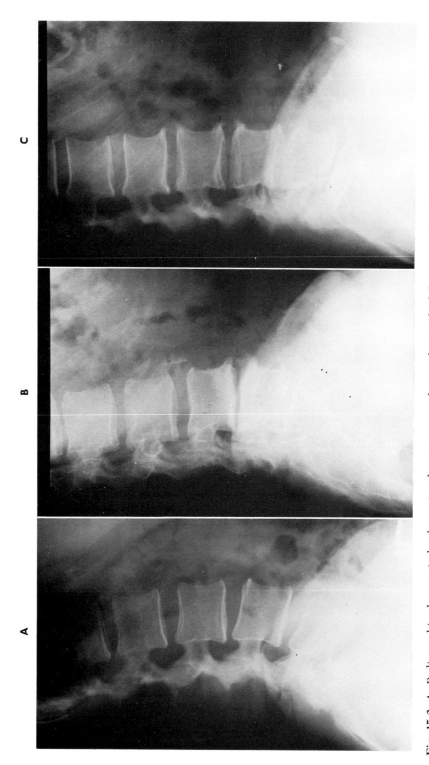

Fig. 15-2. A, Radiographic changes in lumbar spine do not necessarily correlate with ability to run long distances. This 72-year-old man has completed 69 marathons. **B,** This 57-year-old man had a significant period of low back disability 10 years before this x-ray study. He has run in 40 marathons in the past 10 years and is having only minimal discomfort. **C,** This 52-year-old man has run in 80 marathons and is essentially asymptomatic.

referred to the gluteal or thigh area or associated with asymmetrical hamstring tightness. Following a modification in the running program, the symptoms often clear without a specific diagnosis being made. In treating lumbar problems the physician must evaluate the entire lower extremity for imbalances or alterations that can be treated or corrected.

DEMANDS ON THE LUMBAR SPINE DURING RUNNING

The lumbar spine is by far the area of greatest disability in the spine related to running. Hyperextension and cyclic loading of the lumbar spine occur as the hind leg trails in the runner. This is aggravating to most causes of lumbar pain and radicular symptoms. The degree of repetitive hyperextension of the lumbar spine during distance running is unparalleled in any other sport in the age group between 30 and 60 years. The low back moves from the flat-backed position as the foot strikes to an extended lordotic position as the trailing leg leaves the ground. Often the more competitive and faster runners have greater extension in the lumbar spine.

STRUCTURAL CHANGES

Structural changes in the lumbar spine, such as scoliosis, increased lordosis, facet tropism, sacralization, and lumbarization of the lower vertebral segments, are usually not the cause of pain in the runner. However, if these structural changes are accompanied by altered flexibility, restricted range of motion, or associated degenerative changes, symptoms related to the aging process may develop that are aggravated by running. If a middle-aged runner with postural insufficiency begins a running program, subtle structural changes in the lumbosacral anatomy may become more symptomatic. Most runners with radiographic structural variations from normal can run without pain or can return to a modified running program. As mentioned previously, attention should be given to leg length discrepancies in this group.

Spondylolysis, a defect of the pars interarticularis that is present on lumbar x-ray films in skeletally mature runners, is usually an incidental finding (Fig. 15-3). The incidence of lumbar pars interarticularis defects among white male runners is 5% to 10%, although this may vary in certain athletic populations and in different ethnic groups.[4,6,8,17] Most lumbar pars interarticularis defects develop during childhood or early adolescence and are unrelated to pain occurring in the adult runner. However, if the pars interarticularis defect is associated with localized vertebral instability (Fig. 15-4) or vertebral slippage (spondylolisthesis), pain may occur. Often in these cases accelerated disc space narrowing takes place at the level of the instability, indicating that it has been present for some time. Commonly, the pain occurs in the disc above the level of instability, and the narrowed disc noted on the x-ray study has stabilized.

Pars interarticularis defects usually do not require permanent restriction from running. Runners with vertebral slippage often are unaware of their spondylolis-

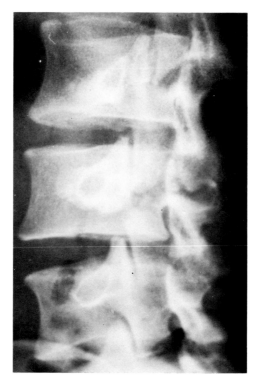

Fig. 15-3. Pars interarticularis defect that was incidental finding in this runner.

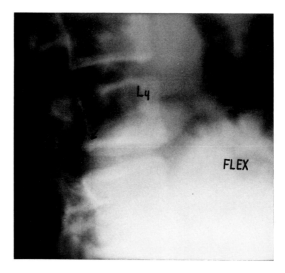

Fig. 15-4. Pars interarticularis defect associated with segmental instability brought out radiographically with forward flexion. Intervertebral disc space was reestablished in extended position.

thesis until it is detected during radiographic examination for a lumbar spine complaint. They are usually able to return to running following conservative treatment. Spondylolysis and spondylolisthesis are not the result of running, but increased demands placed on the lumbar spine, particularly the repetitive extension of the lumbar spine associated with running, may aggravate these conditions. While most low back problems of this type resolve following a period of rest, surgical intervention may be necessary. This is particularly true for patients with painful segmental instability.

INFLAMMATORY CONNECTIVE TISSUE DISEASE

Runners may have manifestations of inflammatory connective tissue disease in the lumbar spine, the sacroiliac joints, or both. These seronegative spondyloarthropathies may be overlooked, particularly in the younger adult age group. The early presentation of spondylitis and its variants should be suspected in the young runner complaining of lumbar spine and sacral discomfort. HLA-B27 tissue typing may be particularly worthwhile in runners with unusual low back pain. Since HLA-B27 can be detected in at least 7% of the normal population, its presence does not establish the diagnosis of inflammatory disease. However, when it is coupled with a dramatic response to anti-inflammatory medication or a positive bone scan, the diagnosis becomes more apparent.

During the examination of the runner, special attention should be given to the sacroiliac joints. The patient may have ankylosing spondylitis or some other variant of Reiter's syndrome. Details concerning other joint involvement, arthritis, urethritis, conjunctivitis, and mucous membrane changes should be obtained. The technetium pyrophosphate bone scan is particularly helpful when early inflammatory changes of the sacroiliac joint are present. The increased bony activity may be seen only on the bone scan. If these changes are part of a self-limited process, they may not be detected on routine x-ray studies or may not develop until years later. They may be associated with periods of disability that respond to rest and anti-inflammatory medication. Usually the athletes are able to continue running. Nonspecific urethritis associated with discomfort in the low back and sacroiliac joints often results in a period of disability, and evaluation of this entity may require an extensive rheumatological and urological workup.

SYMPTOMATIC LUMBAR DISC DISEASE

The role of the intervertebral disc in low back pain is difficult to evaluate. Since the cause of discogenic pain is unknown, most runners with low back pain receive only symptomatic treatment. The low back pain associated with sciatica, which is referred pain in the distribution of the sciatic nerve (dermatomal pain), is usually related to a disc protrusion or rupture. Although degenerative disc disease is extremely common in adults and can even occur in children, only a small number of runners are restricted from running because of diagnosed lumbar disc disease. In a series of 1077 consecutive patients with running injuries only 11 had sciatica.

These runners recovered without surgical intervention and returned to their running programs. The fourth and fifth lumbar discs are the most commonly affected, although in the runner a higher disc must not be overlooked.[7] The sciatic nerve arises from the fourth and fifth lumbar and first, second, and third sacral roots. The pain is typically referred, centered in the lumbar area and radiating into the buttocks, the posterior thigh, the calf, and commonly even the foot. Many runners with sciatica have numbness, tingling, and even weakness in their lower extremities after running. The amount of disability from a ruptured disc depends on several factors, including the size of the bony neural canal, the amount of disc material extravasated, the time during which the pressure has been applied to the nerve, and the patient's response to pain and irritation of a nerve root.

The more degenerative arthritic changes associated with nerve foramina encroachment and spinal stenosis may result in a mild cauda equina syndrome in the older runner. This should not be confused with a vascular problem. The symptoms may be pain and fatigability in the lower extremity with prolonged running. This is an infrequent problem because most people with this advanced degree of degenerative lumbar change have too much pain to carry out prolonged running.

REHABILITATION

Most conservative programs for treating acute disc problems associated with radicular pain are based on rest and antilordotic exercises and positioning. Because of the aggravating effects of repetitive hyperextension, runners with intense acute low back pain who are interested in rapid recovery should consider a period of bed rest. Runners generally do not respond favorably to this suggestion, although if they understand the value of bed rest in their ultimate return to running, they may pay considerably more attention. Traction and analgesics may be prescribed as necessary. The use of anti-inflammatory medication and muscle relaxants should be individualized. A period of controlled rest with a significant reduction in mileage and restriction of other activities can be tried in mild cases.[12] Abdominal exercises and antilordotic positioning for the lumbar spine should be included. The simple use of heat and relaxation techniques may also be tried.

A lumbar epidural cortisone injection has shown some success in runners who have radicular symptoms that persist 2 to 3 weeks or longer and who do not respond to rest (Fig. 15-5). Just one injection may significantly reduce radicular pain and hasten the ability to resume running. The lumbar epidural cortisone injection, along with restricted mileage, flexion exercises, and gradual resumption of the running program, has been successful in about 40% of the athletes in whom we have used it.[12,14] Because of its longer-lasting epidural effects, methylprednisolone acetate (Depo-Medrol) is preferred to the shorter-acting water-soluble suspensions.

Intradiscal cortisone injection has not been beneficial in any of the runners we have treated, and our experience with the lumbar facet injection has been limited. The diagnosis of lumbar facet syndrome is difficult to establish. Some runners have symptoms believed to be related to impingement of the facets from repetitive hy-

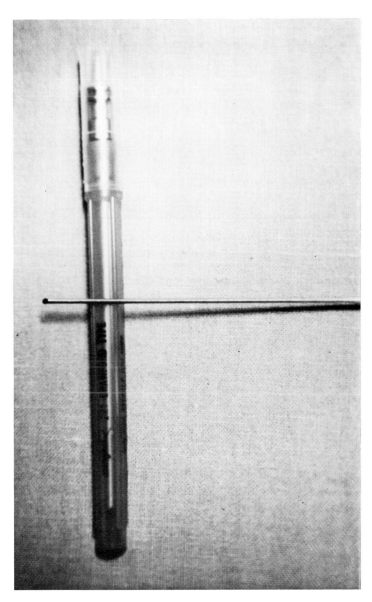

Fig. 15-5. Epidural needle with short beveled point makes it easier to enter epidural space without penetrating dura.

perextension of the lumbar spine during the running gait. If a facet injection is indicated, positioning the needle in the facet joint usually requires image intensification control and may be aided by obtaining a facet arthrogram before the injection. Facet injection has been reported to be beneficial in some patient populations, but no reports establishing its success in runners are available.

Active or passive mobilization (manipulation) of the lumbar spine may be effective in localized lumbar spine problems in distance runners. It can be performed by the physician, by a therapist, or by other persons trained in mobilization techniques. Often mobilization provides only 2 to 3 hours of relief. On occasion, mobilization results in dramatic relief, but in these cases it is usually coupled with additional treatments.

The efficacy of transelectrical nerve stimulation (TENS) in the distance runner is limited. This noninvasive technique may produce temporary analgesia while the underlying process heals. It should not be used to increase the pain tolerance for prolonged training. Most runners respond to rest with or without TENS.

Corsets and antilordotic braces are of little value in the runner unless used during the acute phase to aid in positioning and in restricting activity for a short time. Wetsuit lumbar binders that increase the local skin temperature may relieve symptoms during running in mild cases of low back discomfort.

Some lumbar pain syndromes are aggravated by activities other than running. The running accounts for only a portion of the disability. For example, a runner may have a job requiring prolonged sitting and repeated bending, lifting, and stooping. Although the running produces the greatest aggravation of the back disability, these activities also cause aggravation. Often an alteration of the entire requirements placed on the back is required if the runner is to continue running. It may be helpful to review lifting habits, bending techniques, getting in and out of chairs and automobiles, sleeping positions and surfaces, and placement of a foot on a short stool if prolonged standing is necessary.

PREVENTION OF LOW BACK PAIN

When prevention of spinal symptoms in the runner is the goal, proper stretching, good muscle balance, correct lifting habits, and good posture are important. To minimize the episodes of back symptoms, the runner should stretch regularly, preferably before and after running. There is always a problem of allotting enough time, but a patient with back problems should definitely make a stretching program a priority. Although most runners take time to stretch the Achilles tendon and the hamstrings, they usually do not work specifically on the spine.

Full range of motion of the lumbar spine is maintained by stretching. Most of all the preferred stretching avoids hyperextension of the lumbar spine. This is particularly important when sit-ups and other calisthenics are done as part of the warm-up and cooling down period. Smith[14] outlined a five-point treatment and prevention program for athletes with low back pain: (1) relief of spasm and pain, (2) stretching, (3) exercise, (4) alteration of the training program, and (5) education to prevent future problems or worsening of the present problem. He believed that since the track athlete runs in a forced extension posture and the extensor musculature is significantly more developed than the flexor musculature, it is important for runners to strengthen the abdominal muscles and flatten the lordosis by doing pelvic tilts, curl-ups, and sit-ups in their routine exercise regimen. Fairbank,

O'Brien, and Davis[3] also believed that the abdomen is physiologically important in the support of the lumbar spine. Although the role of exercise in the management of low back pain remains controversial,[2] we prefer to exercise the abdominal musculature and hip flexors as well as the spine. Slow progression of training done in a painless fashion is important if the body is to return to full function.

Lumbar surgery in the runner can be quite successful. We are aware of 12 runners who have returned to marathon running after one-level or multiple-level disc surgery and lumbar spine fusions. However, not all runners are able to run a marathon after lumbar spine surgery. If there is incomplete recovery or resolution of the pain problem following surgery, with associated chronic neural changes, the runner may not be able to continue with a running program. Swimming or bicycling may become a substitute for this individual. It is a popular misconception that a patient who has had lumbar spine surgery is precluded from future running. There is no conclusive evidence that a pain-free spine will undergo more rapid degeneration with running. Runners who have had a disabling back condition of long duration, with or without surgery, are likely to have recurrent episodes of back disability whether they run or not.

Fortunately for the runner, spinal disorders usually respond to conservative treatment and the runner is able to return to unlimited mileage. To minimize spine problems, the runner should maintain flexibility in the spine, use good lifting habits, and be willing to respect warning pains. Running, with its demands of repetitive range of motion of the lumbar spine, particularly the increasing lordosis related to the trailing leg, may be more than certain spines can tolerate. Tolerance is highly individualized, and each patient needs an individual evaluation and interpretation.

SUMMARY

1. Restricting lumbar pain syndromes are uncommon in the runner.

2. A temporary period of rest and mileage restriction during disability is usually the best and most effective treatment of lumbar spine problems. The majority of runners return to running with a satisfactory resolution of the problem.

3. Degenerative changes in the lumbar spine associated with the repetitive hyperextension demands of running may preclude a few runners from running. These processes are usually not the result of running but have been aggravated by running. These individuals should be directed to endurance events that do not aggravate their underlying degenerative process.

4. Lumbar surgery is not usually performed in the runner, but if it is necessary, it does not necessarily preclude a return to a running program.

5. Selective surgery or injections may in certain instances prolong the years of participation in running.

REFERENCES

1. Aggrawal, M.D., and others: A study of changes in the spine in weightlifters and other athletes, Br. J. Sports Med. **13**:58, 1979.
2. Davies, J.E., Gibson, T., and Tester, L.: The value of exercise in the treatment of low back pain, Rheumatol. Rehabil. **18**:243, 1979.

3. Fairbank, J.C., O'Brien, D.P., and Davis, P.R.: Intraabdominal pressure and low back pain (letter), Lancet **1:**1353, 1979.
4. Guten, G.: Herniated lumbar disk associated with running: a review of 10 cases, Am. J. Sports Med. **9:**155, 1981.
5. Harris, W.D.: The lower back in sports medicine, J. Arkansas Med. Soc. **74:**377, 1978.
6. Jackson, D.W., Wiltse, L.L., and Cirincione, R.J.: Spondylolysis in the female gymnast, Clin. Orthop. **117:**68, 1976.
7. Jackson, D.W., Rettig, A., and Wiltse, L.L.: Epidural cortisone injections in the young athletic adult, Am. J. Sports Med. **8:**239, 1980.
8. Jackson, D.W., Wiltse, L.L., and Dingeman, R.: Sub-roentgenographic stress reactions of the posterior elements in young athletes, Am. J. Sports Med. **9:**304, 1981.
9. Pagliano, J.W., and Jackson, D.W.: The ultimate study of running injuries, Runner's World **15:**42, 1980.
10. Palmer, H.: Pain maps in the differential diagnosis of psychosomatic disorders, Med. Press **454:**458, 1960.
11. Ransford, A.O., Cairs, D., and Mooney, V.: The pain drawing as an aid to psychologic evaluation of the patient with low back pain, Spine **1:**127, 1976.
12. Rettig, A., and others: The epidural venogram as a diagnostic procedure in the young athlete with symptoms of lumbar disc disease, Am. J. Sports Med. **5:**158, 1977.
13. Slocum, D.B., and James, S.L.: Biomechanics of running, J.A.M.A. **205:**721, 1968.
14. Smith, C.: Physical management of muscular low back pain in the athlete, Can. Med. Assoc. J. **117:**632, 1977.
15. Stanish, W.: Low back pain in middle-aged athletes, Am. J. Sports Med. **6:**367, 1979.
16. Sutker, A., and Jackson, D.W.: Roentgenographic changes in the lumbar spine in marathon runners. (In press.)
17. Wiltse, L.L., Widell, E.H., and Jackson, D.W.: Fatigue fracture: the basic lesion in isthmic spondylolisthesis, J. Bone Joint Surg. **57A:**17, 1975.

16. Is medial lower leg pain (shin splint) a chronic compartment syndrome?

Richard Wallensten
Ejnar Eriksson

Recurrent pain in the anterior tibial muscle compartment is a well-known entity among athletes. It is usually produced by exercise and relieved by rest. The chronic form has been well described by several investigators.[3-5,12,13] They have shown the pain to be associated with an increase in intramuscular pressure in the compartment, creating a circulatory disturbance with muscle ischemia and delayed venous outflow.[12] It is thought that the tight fascial lining of the muscle compartment is sometimes too rigid to permit swelling of the muscles during exercise,[17] thus causing the increase in pressure.

A more common problem associated with exercise is pain along the medial border of the tibia (medial tibial syndrome or shin splint). Orava[8] reported an incidence of 9.4% in 1179 patients at a sports medicine clinic. The pain starts after exercise and is usually localized between the middle and lower thirds of the tibia. It is often not relieved immediately with rest but can persist for hours and sometimes even days. It has been suggested that this is also a compartment syndrome because of the nature of the symptoms and because they are relieved by surgical release of the fascia from the tibia at the site of pain.[9,10] Moreover, Puranen and Alvaikko[10] found a moderate increase in intramuscular pressure in the deep posterior muscle compartment after exercise. D'Ambrosia and co-workers[1] made pressure measurements in the lower leg at rest in 14 patients. The pressure in the anterior tibial compartment was normal in all 14. The intramuscular pressure in the deep posterior compartment was measured in only three athletes and was found to be normal in all three.

Stress fractures are another reason for lower leg pain in the athlete.[2,16] Devas[2] found 16 such fractures in an unspecified number of athletes with shin splints.

To find out whether lower leg pain after exercise is a chronic compartment syndrome, we examined athletes with lower leg pain referred to us at the Karolinska Hospital in Stockholm.

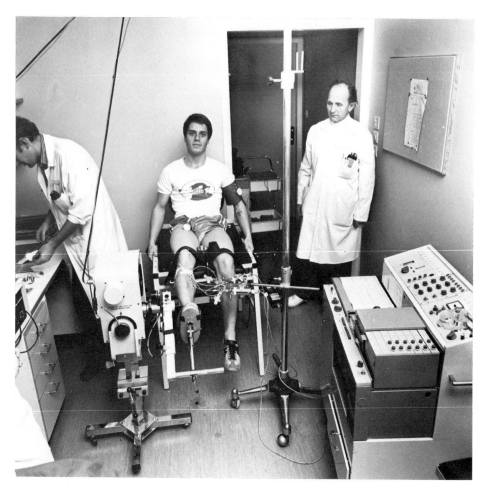

Fig. 16-1. Test model with catheters in place and patient exercising on Cybex dynamometer while pressures are being recorded.

MATERIAL AND METHODS

We examined seven athletes with chronic pain along the medial border of the tibia after exercise and three with chronic pain in the anterior tibial compartment after exercise. All had previous x-ray examination of the lower legs and isotope bone scanning with technetium 99m to exclude stress fractures. Intramuscular pressure was measured with a wick catheter[7] made using a 3-0 Dexone thread pulled into the tip of an epidural catheter (Portex clear epidural cannula, 16 gauge) with the aid of a 6-0 Prolene thread. The wick catheter was connected to a capacitative transducer, and the pressure was recorded on a 6-0 channel Mingograph (Siemens Elema). Wick catheters were introduced percutaneously into the anterior tibial and deep posterior muscle compartments for simultaneous recordings.

Ankle motion

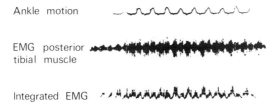

EMG posterior
tibial muscle

Integrated EMG

Fig. 16-2. Electromyographic (EMG) registrations from deep posterior muscle compartment during exercise. Top registration shows ankle motion on dynamometer, middle registration the ordinary EMG, and bottom registration the integrated EMG.

Pressure was recorded before, during, and after exercise. The exercise consisted of ankle flexion and extension in an isokinetic dynamometer (Cybex II, Lumex Corp.) at an angular velocity of 45 degrees/sec. The experimental setup is shown in Fig. 16-1. The subjects exercised with maximum strength until pain in the lower leg forced them to stop. They described this pain as the same as when running.

Previous electromyographic studies with needle electrodes in the anterior and deep posterior compartments had shown these muscles to be engaged during this exercise (Fig. 16-2).

After the pressure investigations, fasciotomy was performed in both groups. This was done subcutaneously through a 4-cm skin incision. The fascia was cut proximally and distally using a Smilie meniscectomy scalpel. The operation was performed as an outpatient procedure, and the patients were allowed immediate weight-bearing and usually resumed training within 2 weeks. In five cases both legs were operated on at the same time.

In 2 to 6 months after surgery, pressure measurements were repeated in exactly the same way as preoperatively.

RESULTS

In the three patients with pain in the anterior tibial compartment, at rest pressures were between 3 and 23 mm Hg. During the first 3-minute period after exercise the pressures rose to between 40 and 90 mm Hg, and they remained elevated more than 6 minutes after exercise (Fig. 16-3). Pressures in the posterior compartment remained normal. Postoperative measurements in the anterior compartment showed resting pressures between 2 and 13 mm Hg and pressures of 11 to 18 mm Hg immediately after exercise and 6 to 18 mm Hg more than 6 minutes after exercise. All three patients had become symptom free.

In the seven patients with medial pain the preoperative resting pressures were between 1 and 16 mm Hg, and in the first 3 minutes after exercise the pressures were between 6 and 22 mm Hg. After more than 6 minutes the pressures were 6 to 13 mm Hg (Fig. 16-4). Postoperative pressures in the deep posterior compartment in these patients were between 0 and 6 mm Hg at rest and 0 to 15 mm Hg in the first 3 minutes after exercise. After 6 minutes they remained the same. No

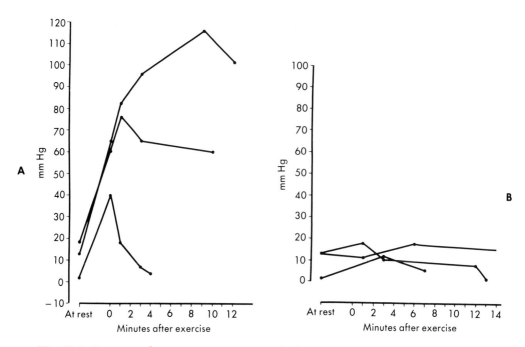

Fig. 16-3. Intramuscular pressure in anterior tibial compartment in patients with anterior tibial pain before and after exercise. **A,** Preoperatively. **B,** After fasciotomy.

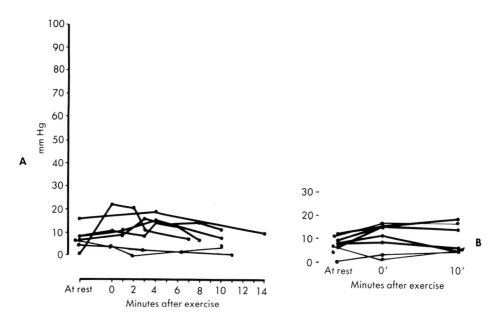

Fig. 16-4. A, Preoperative intramuscular pressure in deep posterior muscle compartment in patients with medial tibial pain before and after exercise. **B,** Intramuscular pressure in deep posterior muscle compartment in healthy subjects before and after exercise.

pressure increase was noted in the anterior compartment. Five of these patients became symptom free after the surgical procedure.

In an unpublished study nine healthy volunteers did exactly the same exercise with the same experimental setup described previously and never had pressures exceeding 25 mm Hg after exercise in either the anterior tibial or the deep posterior muscle compartment.[15] Within 2 minutes after exercise the pressures always returned to the normal resting values of 1 to 7 mm Hg (see Fig. 16-4). In the same study intramuscular pressures in the anterior tibial compartment were normal about 15 minutes after a marathon race in 18 runners, as were the pressures measured in 19 cross-country skiers after an 85-km race.

DISCUSSION

Our results show that the patients with pain in the anterior tibial compartment after exercise had a true compartmental syndrome as described by Reneman.[12] That is, the intramuscular pressure was elevated to a level at which it exceeded the capillary blood pressure, thus causing ischemia. This high pressure only slowly normalized after exercise. Fasciotomy relieved the clinical symptoms in these patients, and postoperatively they did not show an abnormal intramuscular pressure increase during or after exercise. The patients with medial pain, on the other hand, did not have increased intramuscular pressure in the deep posterior compartment even when in pain. The postoperative pressure measurements in these patients were no different from the preoperative determinations. Puranen and Alavaikko[10] have recently reported a moderate pressure increase in the deep posterior compartment in 14 athletes with medial pain. They recorded pressure while the subjects were running in place for 5 minutes. However, the pressure increase did not provoke pain.

Before using our present test model, we tried measuring intramuscular pressures while patients were running on a treadmill or in the corridors of the hospital. This test situation did not work because running on the treadmill was different from running outdoors and provoked only tiredness rather than pain. Furthermore, there were technical problems with the catheters when the subjects were running.

Our failure to find increased intramuscular pressure in the deep posterior compartment in patients with medial tibial pain is consistent with the report of Mubarak,[6] who found a mean after-exercise pressure of 10 mm Hg in 32 patients.

In another study we analyzed percutaneous muscle biopsy specimens from patients with medial and anterolateral lower leg pain.[14] In patients with pain in the anterior tibial muscle compartment we found an after-exercise rise in lactate concentration that was parallel to the rise in intramuscular pressure. This increase in lactate disappeared after fasciotomy. Patients with the medial tibial syndrome did not have any increase in the muscle lactate concentration after exercise, although pain was present.

CONCLUSION

We have found no evidence that medial lower leg pain produced by exercise is due to an increase in compartmental pressure in the deep posterior muscle compartment. That fasciotomy relieves this pain may be due to release of the fascia from the periosteum where they come together on the medial tibial margin. An inflammatory reaction may occur in cases of medial lower leg pain. This would explain the increase in isotope uptake described by Westlin.[16] Rasmussen and Sköld[11] in a randomized study of the effect of ultrasonography and placebo treatment on medial tibial pain found that both treatments were effective. Some of the relief of symptoms following surgery may therefore be a placebo effect. Medial tibial pain after exercise is probably mechanical in origin or an overstrain inflammation process. Further studies are needed.

REFERENCES

1. D'Ambrosia, R.D., and others: Interstitial pressure measurements in the anterior and posterior compartments in athletes with shin splints, Am. J. Sports Med. **5:**127, 1977.
2. Devas, M.B.: Stress fractures of the tibia in athletes or "shin soreness," J. Bone Joint Surg. **40B:**227, 1958.
3. French, E.B., and Price, W.H.: Anterior tibial pain, Br. Med. J. **2:**1290, 1962.
4. Leach, R.E., Hammond, G., and Stryker, W.: Anterior tibial compartment syndrome: acute and chronic, J. Bone Joint Surg. **49A:**451, 1967.
5. Mavor, G.E.: The anterior tibial syndrome, J. Bone Joint Surg. **38B:**513, 1956.
6. Mubarak, S.J.: Clinical wick catheter technique. In Hargens, A.: Tissue fluid pressure and composition, Baltimore, 1981, The Williams & Wilkins Co.
7. Mubarak, S.J., and others: The wick catheter technique for measurement of intramuscular pressure: a new research and clinical tool, J. Bone Joint Surg. **58A:**1016, 1976.
8. Orava, S.: Exertion injuries due to sports and physical exercise: a clinical and statistical study of nontraumatic overuse injuries of the musculoskeletal system of athletes and keep-fit athletes, Scientific thesis, Turku, Finland, 1980.
9. Puranen, J.: The medial tibial syndrome: exercise ischemia in the medial fascial compartment of the leg, J. Bone Joint Surg. **56B:**712, 1974.
10. Puranen, J., and Alavaikko, A.: Intracompartmental pressure increase on exertion in patients with chronic compartment syndrome in the leg, J. Bone Joint Surg. **63A:**1304, 1981.
11. Rasmussen, E., and Sköld, P.: Hjälper ultraljud mot benhinneinflammation? (Does ultrasound cure shin splint?), Idrottsmedicin **1:**10, 1981.
12. Reneman, R.S.: The anterior and the lateral compartmental syndrome of the leg due to intensive use of muscles, Clin. Orthop. Rel. Res. **113:**69, 1975.
13. Snook, G.A.: Intermittent claudication in athletes, J. Sports Med. **3:**71, 1975.
14. Wallensten, R.: Medial lower leg pain after exercise: a chronic compartment syndrome? Exerc. Sport Biol. (In press.)
15. Wallensten, R., and Eklund, B.: Intramuscular pressures and exercise. (In press.)
16. Westlin, M.E.: Stressfrakturer (Stress fractures), Läkartidningen **74:**123, 1977.
17. Wiklund, P.E.: Closed compartment syndrom i nedre extremiteten (Closed compartment syndrome of the leg), Läkartidningen **74:**121, 1977.

17. Exertional compartment syndromes

Scott Mubarak
Alan Hargens

A compartment syndrome results when increased tissue fluid pressure in a closed fascial compartment compromises the circulation to the nerves and muscles within the involved compartment. The initial injury causes hemorrhage or edema, or both, to accumulate in the compartment. The noncompliance of the compartment's fascial boundaries causes an increase in intramuscular fluid pressure that in turn produces ischemia. Without immediate decompression of the compartment there may be permanent damage to the muscles and nerves in the compartment. The syndrome is most commonly caused by a fracture, severe contusion, or postischemic swelling. Rarely, strenuous exercise may initiate compartment syndromes.

The exercise-initiated compartment syndromes are divided into two types on the basis of clinical findings and reversibility. An acute syndrome exists when intramuscular pressure is elevated to a level and duration such that immediate decompression is necessary to prevent intracompartmental necrosis. The clinical findings, natural history, and treatment are the same as in a compartment syndrome initiated by a fracture or contusion, but the event occurs following intense use of muscles and there is no external trauma. The second type, the chronic or recurrent compartment syndrome, exists when exercise raises the intramuscular pressure sufficiently to produce small vessel compromise and therefore ischemia, pain, and (rarely) neurological deficit. These symptoms disappear when the activity is stopped and reappear during the next period of exercise. However, if the exercise is continued, a chronic compartment syndrome may proceed to an acute syndrome requiring emergency surgical decompression. An example is the military recruit who exercises under duress beyond his limits of pain tolerance.

HISTORY

The first description of anterior compartment syndrome initiated by exertion was probably that by Dr. Edward Wilson, the medical officer on Captain R.F. Scott's ill-fated race to the South Pole.[14] On the return trip from the Pole, Dr. Wilson began experiencing severe pain and swelling in the area of the anterior compartment, which he accurately described in his diary. In a lecture 31 years later in 1943, Vogt[54] described a case of ischemic muscle necrosis following marching. In 1944 Horn[23] reported two more cases, one involving the anterior and lateral compartment and the other an isolated case of the anterior compartment. That same year, Sirbu, Murphy, and White[49] described a case of the anterior compartment syndrome resulting from a long march. Two cases of the acute syndrome with isolated lateral compartment involvement[6] and one case involving the superficial posterior compartment[38] have also been reported.

In 1956 Mavor[32] first described the chronic or recurrent form of the anterior exertional compartment syndrome. His patient had recurring pain in the anterior compartment associated with numbness and muscle hernia. Fasciotomy relieved this problem. The pressure studies of French and Price[15] confirmed the existence of the chronic syndrome, which had previously been questioned by others.[19,20] Reneman,[44] in his monograph on this subject, reported more than 61 chronic cases, also with pressure documentation.

A chronic form involving other compartments of the leg has been described, although tissue pressure documentation is lacking. Reneman[44] reported seven cases of the chronic syndrome involving both the lateral and anterior compartments. Kirby[26] described a patient with bilateral chronic superficial posterior compartment syndromes; this patient's symptoms were relieved by fasciotomies. Three additional cases of chronic syndromes in the superficial posterior compartment were reported by Snook.[51] Eleven cases of exertional syndromes involving the deep posterior tibial compartment were reported by Puranen.[42]

Isolated involvement of the second interosseous compartment of the hand[43] and the volar compartment of the forearm[52] has also been documented.

PATHOGENESIS

Elevated intramuscular pressure is the immediate cause of muscle and nerve ischemia in exertional compartment syndromes.[15,35,45] The factors responsible for the elevation of intramuscular pressure in certain individuals following exercise remain speculative. The pressure rises in the compartment owing to the limitation of compartment size and the increase in the compartment volume. The following are the probable factors in the pathogenesis of the exertional compartment syndrome:

    I. Limited compartment size (thickened fascia)
    II. Increased volume of compartment contents
        A. Acute
            1. Muscle swelling owing to increased capillary permeability and intracellular edema
            2. Restricted venous or lymphatic outflow
            3. Hemorrhage owing to torn muscle fibers
        B. Chronic (muscle hypertrophy)

During exercise two interesting phenomena occur (Fig. 17-1). First, during a strong isometric or isotonic contraction, intramuscular pressure rises sufficiently to render the muscle ischemic while the contraction is maintained. This fact has been noted by a number of authors using a variety of indirect methods of estimating

NORMAL　　　　　CHRONIC
EXERCISE　　　　　ACUTE
EXERCISE

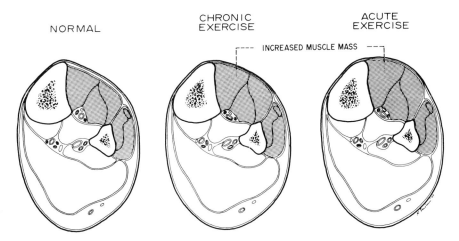

Fig. 17-1. Cross-section through midportion of right leg demonstrating increased volume of anterior compartment contents with chronic exercise owing to muscle hypertrophy *(center)* and with acute exercise owing to increased capillary permeability, intracellular and extracellular edema, and hemorrhage *(right)*. (From Mubarak, S.J., and Hargens, A.R.: Compartment syndromes and Volkmann's contracture, Philadelphia, 1981, W.B. Saunders Co.)

tissue pressure,* and it has been confirmed in our laboratory by direct measurement of the muscle during contraction using the wick catheter.[36,39] During a muscle contraction the pressure rises acutely, probably both by mechanical means and as a result of cessation of blood flow from the muscle.

Second, with prolonged exercise, muscle increases acutely in bulk by as much as 20%.[58] Linge[30] demonstrated acute hypertrophy in untrained rats after 5 hours of exercise. Gershuni and associates[17] used ultrasound scanning of the anterior compartment to demonstrate an acute increase in muscle volume with exercise in normal subjects. These findings are probably due to increased capillary permeability resulting in fluid accumulation in both the intracellular and extracellular spaces. Other possibilities have been suggested to account for the volume increase in the compartment of subjects under exercise conditions (Fig. 17-1). Anomalies of venous or lymphatic return may exist in patients with the chronic syndrome.[44] Unaccustomed exercise may lead to hemorrhage from torn muscle fibers as an additional source of fluid accumulation.[8,41] In the chronic syndrome, muscle hypertrophy occurs with repeated exercise or conditioning. Whatever the cause, the pressure rise is well documented, and therefore fluid must accumulate in the compartments' interstitial spaces.

ACUTE EXERTIONAL COMPARTMENT SYNDROME
Clinical presentation

Excessive use of muscles as a cause of an acute compartment syndrome is extremely uncommon. Fewer than 100 cases are documented in the literature, and

*References 2-4, 18, 22, 27, 55.

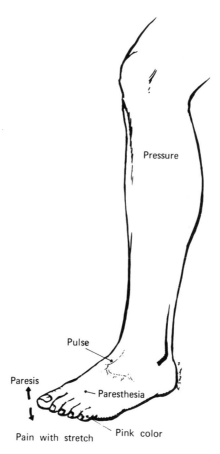

Fig. 17-2. Early findings of acute compartment syndrome illustrated in anterior compartment. (From Mubarak, S.J., and others: Pressure measurement with the wick catheter. In Practice of Surgery, Hagerstown, Md., 1978, Harper & Row, Publishers.)

in the past 6 years in our study of over 100 patients with acute syndromes, only two cases have been initiated by exercise. The reported cases of acute exertional compartment syndromes involved the leg, usually the anterior compartment.

The majority of reported cases of the acute syndrome developed in patients performing unaccustomed tasks such as forced marches or prolonged runs. Some patients had symptoms of a chronic compartment syndrome for months before the acute episode (17% in Reneman's series).[45] The initial symptom of the acute compartment syndrome is severe pain over the involved compartment. The pain is initiated during the exercise or develops within 12 hours after the exercise. As the pain increases, numbness and weakness are noted and medical attention is sought.

The clinical findings in acute compartment syndromes initiated by exertion are identical to those in an acute syndrome of any cause (Fig. 17-2). Increased tension (pressure) and pain occur over the involved compartment or compartments.

Stretching the involved muscles of the compartment exacerbates this pain. Muscle weakness (paresis) and a sensory deficit are often present. Capillary fill and the pedal pulses (dorsalis pedis and posterior tibial) are routinely intact, although palpation may be difficult because of ankle and foot edema. Even though intramuscular pressure may be high enough to cause ischemia to muscle and nerve, it is rarely high enough to occlude a major artery.

Laboratory investigations

Tissue pressure measurement is the best objective test for determining the need for fasciotomy. For the past 7 years we have employed the wick and slit catheter techniques for this purpose.[35,47] These techniques provide an accurate and reproducible means of determining tissue pressure under equilibrium conditions. Other techniques have also been found to be valuable in the diagnosis of acute compartment syndromes.[7,31,56] If the intramuscular pressures are greater than 30 mm Hg (normal is 0 to 8 mm Hg) in a normotensive patient with the appropriate clinical manifestations, surgical decompression should be performed immediately.[21,38]

If there is a question of a possible coexistent arterial injury with the compartment syndrome, arteriography and Doppler studies should be used. When only a compartment syndrome is present, arteriography shows small vessel (arteriolar) cutoff created by the pressure elevations.

Differential diagnosis

In a patient with swelling and neurovascular deficit the acute compartment syndrome must be differentiated from a direct nerve contusion (neurapraxia) and an arterial injury. Since these may coexist with an acute compartment syndrome, tissue pressure measurement and arteriography are extremely important in the diagnosis. Problems such as a large subcutaneous hematoma or an abscess may be manifested by swelling and severe pain; however, without a neurological deficit they are usually easily differentiated from a compartment syndrome.

Treatment

As for any acute compartment syndrome, the treatment is immediate surgical decompression. For this we have employed the double incision technique, using one or both incisions as necessary to decompress the involved compartments. The details of this technique are described elsewhere.[34] The wounds are left open and the limb is splinted. In 5 to 7 days delayed primary closure or skin grafting is performed.

CHRONIC OR RECURRENT EXERTIONAL COMPARTMENT SYNDROME
Clinical presentation

The terminology for the chronic form of the exertional compartment syndrome is somewhat confusing. Veith, Matsen, and Newell[53] have used the term "recurrent compartmental syndrome," whereas Rorabeck[46] prefers the adjective "subacute." We prefer the term "chronic compartment syndrome."

The chronic syndrome is much more common than the acute form. Reneman[45] has reported the largest series (61 cases), nearly all of which involved only the anterior compartment. The symptoms were bilateral in 95% of his patients and in about 75% of ours.[34] The majority of patients were males.

In most cases the patient reports recurrent pain over the anterior or lateral compartment area that is initiated by exercise and has been present for months. The exercise may vary from a prolonged walk or march to a marathon run. For a given patient the onset of the pain is reproducible for a specific speed and distance or activity. Usually the patient must discontinue his run and rest for a few minutes. However, this varies; some individuals can continue to run at a reduced speed, whereas others who discontinue their exercise immediately may be bothered by symptoms for hours.

The pain is described as a feeling of pressure, aching, cramping, or a stabbing sensation over the anterior compartment. Associated symptoms including numbness on the dorsum of the foot, weakness, or footdrop may occasionally be present.

Physical examination before exercise shows few abnormalities. Neurocirculatory findings are normal. Usually the muscles are well developed in all compartments.

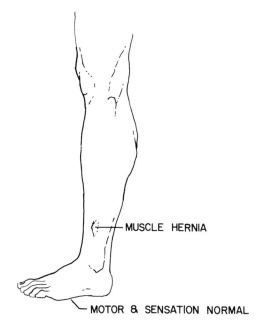

MUSCLE HERNIA

MOTOR & SENSATION NORMAL

Fig. 17-3. Muscle hernias are commonly associated with chronic exertional compartment syndromes, and neurologic examination is usually normal. (From Mubarak, S.J., and Hargens, A.R.: Compartment syndromes and Volkmann's contracture, Philadelphia, 1981, W.B. Saunders Co.)

It is best to ask the patient to perform the run or exercise that initiates the problem. After exercise a sensation of increased fullness over the anterior compartment may be noted, but the neurocirculatory status usually remains normal. Hypesthesia is occasionally found on the dorsum of the foot. Diminished pedal pulses after exercise warrant further workup of the vascular system.

Muscle hernias, noted in 60% of Reneman's patients,[45] may be more obvious clinically after exercise. We have encountered these fascial defects much less fre-

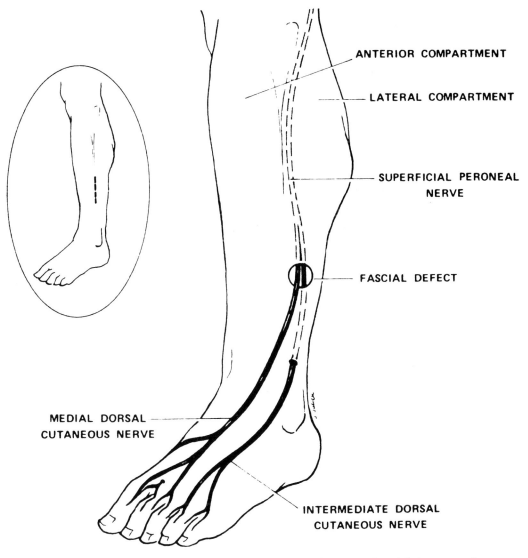

ANTERIOR COMPARTMENT

LATERAL COMPARTMENT

SUPERFICIAL PERONEAL NERVE

FASCIAL DEFECT

MEDIAL DORSAL CUTANEOUS NERVE

INTERMEDIATE DORSAL CUTANEOUS NERVE

Fig. 17-4. Relationship of branches of superficial peroneal nerve to fascial defect. Inset shows skin incision used for fasciotomy in presence of fascial defect. (From Garfin, S., and others: J. Bone Joint Surg. **59:**404, 1977.)

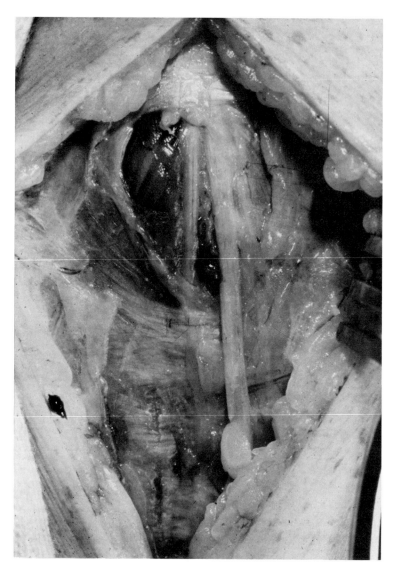

Fig. 17-5. Intraoperative photograph of fascial defect in lower one third of patient's right leg. Medial dorsal cutaneous nerve is to right exiting defect, and intermediate dorsal cutaneous nerve is to left.

quently (30%).[34] Most are located in the lower one third of the leg overlying the anterior intermuscular septum between the anterior and lateral compartments (Fig. 17-3). In this location the fascial defect may represent an enlargement of the orifice through which a branch of the superficial peroneal nerve (medial dorsal cutaneous nerve) exits the lateral compartment. This situation was present in three of our patients. The muscle herniation may cause superficial peroneal nerve irritation and even neuroma formation (Figs. 17-4 and 17-5).[16,44]

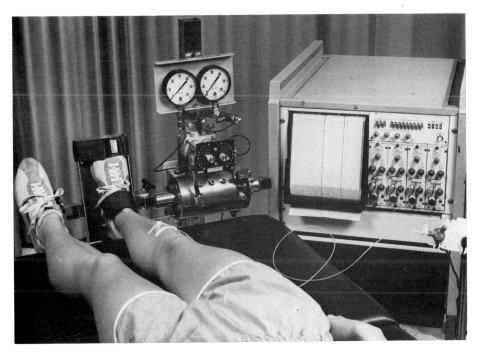

Fig. 17-6. Wick catheter has been inserted into right anterior compartment of patient with suspected chronic compartment syndrome. Foot is attached to isokinetic exerciser. Intracompartmental pressures are continuously recorded by patient's wick catheter connected to pressure transducer and strip recorder. (From Mubarak, S.J., and Hargens, A.R.: Compartment syndromes and Volkmann's contracture, Philadelphia, 1981, W.B. Saunders Co.)

Laboratory investigations

Tissue pressure measurement. The study of chronic syndromes using the needle technique was first employed by French and Price[15] in 1962. Reneman,[44] using the same technique, investigated a large number of patients. He found that the intramuscular pressures at rest, immediately after exercise, and at 6 minutes after exercise exceeded normal values in control subjects of comparable age. He could not measure the pressures continuously during exercise with this technique.

Because of the advantage of continuous monitoring during the exercise, we prefer the wick or slit catheter techniques.[36,47] Using these techniques, we have also observed differences in pressure between normal subjects and patients with the chronic syndrome. The catheter is inserted into the involved compartment under sterile conditions and local anesthesia. It is taped in position, and pressure measurements are determined during complete rest in the supine position. The subject's foot is then attached to a isokinetic exerciser (Orthotron, Lumex Corp.) using the foot attachment apparatus (Fig. 17-6). A standard setting is used for all patients. The subject is instructed to perform dorsiflexion and plantar flexion of the foot once every 2 seconds until pain or fatigue forces him to stop. The pressures are continuously recorded by the catheter connected to a pressure transducer and strip recorder. We have found this method of exercise to give the most standard results, although on occasion we have employed a treadmill or had the patient run his usual distance to initiate the pain. Reinsertion of the wick or slit catheter in these circumstances must be rapid because the intramuscular pressures fall quickly after exercise.

The mean resting pressure of the anterior compartment of normal subjects in the supine position is 4 ± 4 mm Hg. During exercise the pressure rises to more than 50 mm Hg. Moreover, intramuscular pressure rises and falls with each muscle contraction and relaxation. When the exercise is terminated because of fatigue or pain, the intramuscular pressure begins to fall. In normal subjects the pressure declines to less than 30 mm Hg immediately, and within 5 minutes it returns to the preexercise rest levels in most cases (Fig. 17-7).

The resting intramuscular pressure is usually greater than 15 mm Hg in patients with the chronic syndrome (Fig. 17-7). During exercise the pressure rises to greater than 75 mm Hg. At times the pressure during exercise may exceed 100 mm Hg.

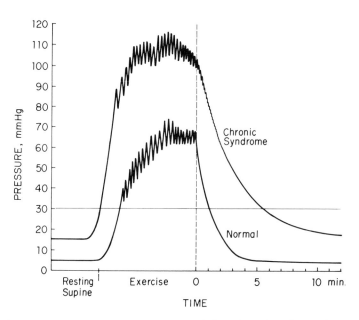

Fig. 17-7. Anterior compartment pressures recorded with wick catheter during exercise of normal subject and patient afflicted with chronic anterior compartment syndrome. Resting pressure of patient with chronic syndrome is greater than that of normal control. During exercise, pressure rises to greater than 75 mm Hg and remains greater than 30 mm Hg for more than 5 minutes in patient with chronic syndrome. (From Mubarak, S.J., and Hargens, A.R.: Compartment syndromes and Volkmann's contracture, Philadelphia, 1981, W.B. Saunders Co.)

At completion of the exercise the intramuscular pressure remains greater than 30 mm Hg for 5 minutes or longer, and usually pain and sometimes paresthesia are present. We have used these findings as our laboratory confirmation of the chronic compartment syndrome. For these patients we recommend fasciotomy, which should normalize both resting and postexercise intramuscular pressure.

Venography. Venography was employed by Reneman[44] in his study of the chronic syndrome. When neither anterior tibial vein filled at 2 to 4 minutes after exercise, he considered this diagnostic of a chronic syndrome. Although this was an interesting investigation, the technique is much more invasive than tissue pressure measurement.

Electromyography and nerve conduction. Leach, Hammond, and Stryker[29] described one patient who demonstrated denervation potentials in the anterior compartment. Reneman[44] used electromyography in five patients. He could demonstrate no abnormality either at rest or during exercise. We agree that electromyography is of little value, although nerve conduction may be helpful if there is a subjective neurological deficit in a patient with a possible chronic compartment syndrome.

Sodium chloride 22 clearance. French and Price[15] and Kennelly and Blumberg[25] demonstrated reduced clearance of sodium chloride 22 after exercise but no change at rest when compared to normal values. We have had no experience with this technique.

Differential diagnosis

Intermittent claudication caused by partial femoral artery obstruction is characterized by symptoms identical to those in the chronic exertional compartment syndrome, but patients with the former tend to be older. The pedal pulses are present when the patient is at rest and disappear with exercise. An arteriogram confirms this diagnosis.

Stress fractures of the tibia or fibula can be diagnosed clinically by noting local tenderness over the bone at the fracture site. Although x-ray findings are initially negative, changes can usually be demonstrated 10 to 14 days after the onset of the pain. A bone scan is usually positive at the onset and may be helpful in the diagnosis.

Tenosynovitis of the dorsiflexors of the foot is characterized by crepitus, erythema, and pain localized to the dorsum of the foot and ankle during movement of the involved tendons.

Cellulitis may initially suggest a compartment syndrome. In most cases the patients are febrile with a loss of function as a result of pain.

Shin splints are usually defined as pain over the anterior compartment associated with activity at the beginning of the sports season after a relatively inactive period.[50] The pain usually clears in about 2 weeks as the athlete becomes conditioned. Reneman[44] believes that shin splints may represent a mild form of the chronic compartment syndrome.

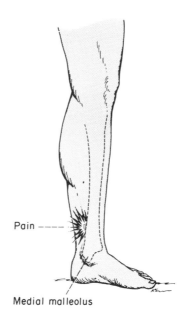

Pain ----

Medial malleolus

Fig. 17-8. Clinical findings of medial tibial syndrome. Patient has localized area of tenderness over posteromedial edge of distal one third of tibia. (From Mubarak, S.J., and Hargens, A.R.: Compartment syndromes and Volkmann's contracture, Philadelphia, 1981, W.B. Saunders Co.)

The medial tibial stress syndrome has been classified by various authors as a stress fracture,[11] a deep posterior compartment syndrome,[42] or a shin splint.[1,24,50] The true cause is unknown. The physical findings are very specific. The patient has a localized area of tenderness over the posteromedial edge of the distal one third of the tibia (Fig. 17-8). This area is often indurated and extremely tender, especially after exertion. Injection of lidocaine into the tender area relieves the pain. Initial x-ray studies are normal. If the duration of the pain exceeds 3 weeks, hypertrophy of the cortex and possibly periosteal new bone formation may be noted. Bone scanning may demonstrate a mild uptake,[34,42] but not as greatly increased as with a stress fracture. Normal tissue pressure measurements of the deep posterior compartment in these patients have been documented by four different investigating teams.[10,12,13,34] The treatment of this entity is in wide dispute. Recommendations include rest,[1] casting,[1] taping,[24] heel pads,[1] anti-inflammatory agents,[1,9] local corticosteroid injection,[24] and fasciotomy.[42]

Treatment

Once the diagnosis of chronic exertional compartment syndrome of the leg has been established on the basis of the history, examination, and pressure measurements, fasciotomy is usually required. However, many patients after hearing the diagnosis and treatment prefer to limit their running or alter their exercise pro-

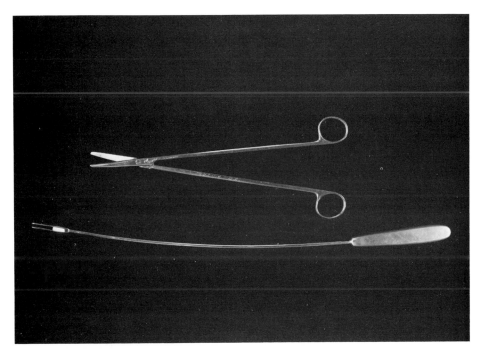

Fig. 17-9. Twelve-inch Metzenbaum scissors and fasciotome. (From Mubarak, S.J., and Hargens, A.R.: Diagnosis and management of compartment syndromes. In AAOS symposium on trauma to the leg and its sequelae, St. Louis, 1981, The C.V. Mosby Co.)

gram. With the chronic compartment syndrome there is not the urgent need for fasciotomy that is present with an acute syndrome. Reneman[45] described 10 patients who declined his recommended surgical decompression and were all symptomatic at 10 to 12 months' follow-up. Most patients who desire to maintain their previous level of jogging or running require fasciotomy.

Mavor[32] was the first to successfully treat a chronic compartment syndrome with fasciotomy. Reneman,[44] who has the greatest experience, uses a blind technique for decompression of the anterior compartment. This technique is not useful in the lateral compartment because of the location of the superficial peroneal nerve. Reneman minimizes the skin incision by using a diathermic wire to burn through the fascia.

We prefer a more direct approach and can accomplish a satisfactory fasciotomy of both the anterior and lateral compartments through a 2-inch skin incision.[34]

The necessary instruments for this procedure include right-angle retractors, a 12-inch Metzenbaum scissors, and/or a fasciotome (Fig. 17-9). We have developed a commercially available fasciotome* modified from the instruments suggested by

*Made by Down Surgical Company, Toronto.

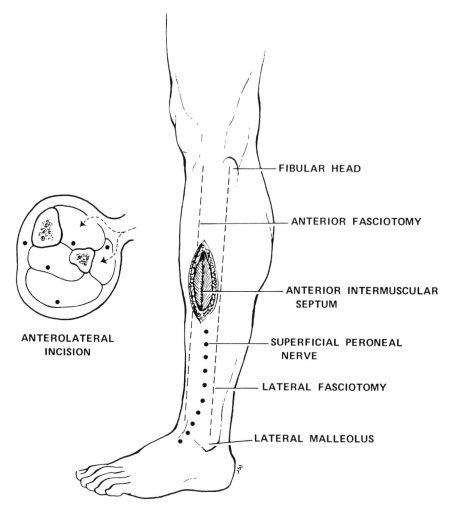

Fig. 17-10. Skin incision used for decompression of anterior and lateral compartments. (From Mubarak, S.J., and Owen, C.A.: J. Bone Joint Surg. **59:**184, 1977.)

others.[5,33,48] The fasciotome is designed to incise the fascia without the need for a long skin incision.

For either anterior or lateral compartment involvement both compartments are decompressed. The skin incision is in the midportion of the leg halfway between the fibula and the anterior portion of the tibial crest. The usual length is 2 inches (Fig. 17-10).

Muscle hernias are frequently noted in the lower one third of the leg in the area overlying the anterior intermuscular septum. In this site one or both sensory branches of the superficial peroneal nerve emerge through the fascia. If a muscle hernia is present, the skin incision should be located over it so that the surgeon can

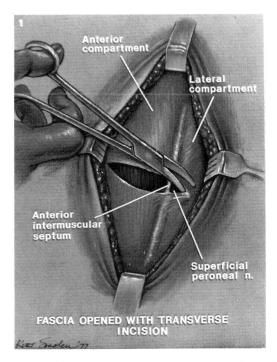

Fig. 17-11. Close-up view of first step in anterolateral incision. (From Mubarak, S.J., and Hargens, A.R.: Diagnosis and management of compartment syndromes. In AAOS symposium on trauma to the leg and its sequelae, St. Louis, 1981, The C.V. Mosby Co.)

explore the fascial defect and identify the superficial peroneal nerve (Fig. 17-4). Through this approach the surgeon can easily decompress both the anterior and lateral compartments. *Closure of a fascial defect is contraindicated because of the risk of precipitating an acute compartment syndrome.**

After the skin incision is made, the edges are undermined proximally and distally to permit wide exposure of the fascia. It should be possible to visualize almost the full extent of the compartment fascia. This is extremely important when using a small incision. A transverse incision is then made through the fascia to identify the anterior intermuscular septum that separates the anterior compartment from the lateral compartment (Fig. 17-11). Identification of this septum is necessary to find the superficial peroneal nerve, which lies in the lateral compartment next to the septum. Using the long Metzenbaum scissors or the fasciotome, the surgeon opens the anterior compartment (Fig. 17-12). Visualization is aided by retraction with the right-angle retractors. Under direct vision the scissors, with the tips open slightly, is pushed distally in the direction of the great toe and proximally toward the patella. If there is any question of whether the tips of the scissors have strayed

---

*References 28, 29, 40, 49, 57.

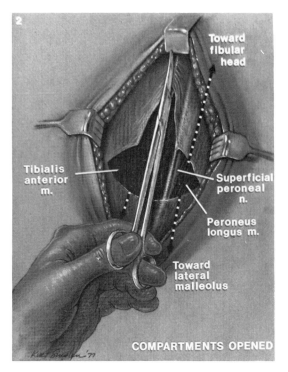

Fig. 17-12. Close-up view of second step in anterolateral incision. (From Mubarak, S.J., and Hargens, A.R.: Diagnosis and management of compartment syndromes. In AAOS symposium on trauma to the leg and its sequelae, St. Louis, 1981, The C.V. Mosby Co.)

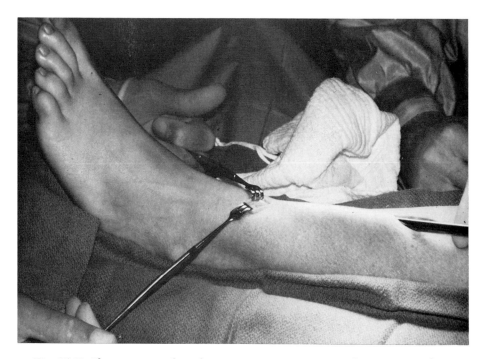

Fig. 17-13. If scissors stray from fascia, accessory incision is made over scissors' tip.

from the fascia, the scissors is left in place and a small incision is made over the tips. If the fasciotomy is incomplete, further release can be performed through this accessory incision (Fig. 17-13).

The lateral compartment fasciotomy is made in line with the fibular shaft (Fig. 17-12). The scissors or fasciotome is directed proximally toward the fibular head and distally toward the lateral malleolus. This produces a fascial incision posterior to the superficial peroneal nerve. The wound is closed with an intradermal running stitch. A light dressing is applied.

The patient is usually discharged on the day after the operation. Light exercises are begun within 10 days and are gradually increased according to the patient's symptoms and clinical course.

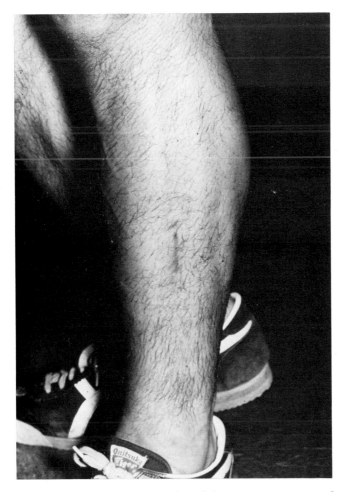

Fig. 17-14. Well-healed scar following anterolateral fasciotomy in runner who had chronic exertional compartment syndrome. (From Mubarak, S.J., and Hargens, A.R.: Compartment syndromes and Volkmann's contracture, Philadelphia, 1981, W.B. Saunders Co.)

Follow-up studies of patients who have had surgical decompression demonstrate a more normal tissue pressure measurement during exercise (Fig. 17-14). In Reneman's patients the pressures at rest and after exercise did not completely return to normal levels.[44] In the few patients we have studied after fasciotomy, the tissue pressure measurements were essentially the same as those of normal runners.

ACKNOWLEDGMENTS

We thank Robbie Davis for her assistance in preparing this manuscript. The research was supported by USPMS grant AM-18824 and the Veterans Administration.

REFERENCES

1. Andrish, J.T., Bergfeld, J.A., and Walheim, J.: A prospective study on the management of shin splints, J. Bone Joint Surg. **56A**:1697, 1974.
2. Anrep, G.V., Blalock, A., and Samaan, A.: The effect of muscular contraction upon blood flow in skeletal muscle, Proc. R. Soc. Lond. (Biol.) **114**:223, 1934.
3. Ashton, H.: The effect of increased tissue pressure on blood flow, Clin. Orthop. **113**:15, 1975.
4. Barcroft, H., and Millen, J.L.E.: The blood flow through muscle during sustained contraction, J. Physiol. **97**:17, 1939.
5. Bate, J.T.: A subcutaneous fasciotome, Clin. Orthop. **83**:235, 1972.
6. Blandy, J.P., and Fuller, R.: March gangrene, J. Bone Joint Surg. **39B**:679, 1957.
7. Brooker, A.R., and Pezeshki, C.: Tissue pressure to evaluate compartmental syndrome, J. Trauma **19**:689, 1979.
8. Carter, A.B., Richards, R.L., and Zachary, R.B.: The anterior tibial syndrome, Lancet **2**:928, 1949.
9. Clement, D.B.: Tibial stress syndrome in athletes, J. Sports Med. **2**:81, 1974.
10. D'Ambrosia, R.D., and others: Interstitial pressure measurements in the anterior and posterior compartments in athletes with shin splints, Am. J. Sports Med. **5**:127, 1977.
11. Devas, M.B.: Stress fractures of the tibia in athletes or "shin soreness," J. Bone Joint Surg. **40B**:227, 1958.
12. Drez, D.: Personal communication, 1981.
13. Eriksson, E., and Wallensten, R.: Can research into muscle morphology and muscle metabolism improve orthopaedic treatment? Proceedings of a meeting of the Western Orthopaedic Association, Las Vegas, Nevada, October 16, 1979.
14. Freedman, B.J.: Dr. Edward Wilson of the Antarctic; a biographical sketch, followed by an inquiry into the nature of his last illness, Proc. R. Soc. Med. **47**:7, 1953.
15. French, E.B., and Price, W.H.: Anterior tibial pain, Br. Med. J. **2**:1290, 1962.
16. Garfin, S.R., Mubarak, S.J., and Owen, C.A.: Exertional anterolateral compartment syndrome, J. Bone Joint Surg. **59A**:404, 1977.
17. Gershuni, D.H., and others: Ultrasound scanning to evaluate the anterior musculofascial compartment of the leg, Orthop. Trans. **5**:293, 1981.
18. Grant, R.T.: Observations on the blood circulation in voluntary muscle in man, Clin. Sci. **3**:157, 1938.
19. Griffiths, D.L.: The anterior tibial syndrome: a chronic form? J. Bone Joint Surg. **38B**:438, 1956.
20. Grunwald, A., and Silberman, Z.: Anterior tibial syndrome, J.A.M.A. **171**:132, 1959.
21. Hargens, A.R., and others: Peripheral nerve conduction block by high muscle compartment pressure, J. Bone Joint Surg. **61A**:192, 1979.
22. Hill, A.V.: The pressure developed in muscle during contraction, J. Physiol. **107**:518, 1948.
23. Horn, C.E.: Acute ischemia of the anterior tibial muscle and the long extensor muscles of the toes, J. Bone Joint Surg. **27A**:615, 1945.
24. Jackson, D.W., and Bailey, D.: Shin splints in the young athlete: a nonspecific diagnosis, Phys. Sportsmed. **3**:45, 1975.
25. Kennelly, B.M., and Blumberg, L.: Bilateral anterior tibial claudication, J.A.M.A. **203**:487, 1968.
26. Kirby, N.G.: Exercise ischemia in the fascial compartment of the soleus, J. Bone Joint Surg. **52B**:738, 1970.
27. Kjellmer, I.: An indirect method for estimating tissue pressure with special reference to tissue pressure in muscle during exercise, Acta Physiol. Scand. **62**:31, 1964.

28. Leach, R.E., Zohn, D.A., and Stryker, W.S.: Anterior tibial compartment syndrome, Arch. Surg. **88**:187, 1964.
29. Leach, R.E., Hammond, G., and Stryker, W.S.: Anterior tibial compartment syndrome: acute and chronic, J. Bone Joint Surg. **49A**:451, 1967.
30. Linge, B. van: Experimentele spierhypertrofie bij de rat, Assen, Netherlands, 1959, Van Garkum.
31. Matsen, F.A., and others: Monitoring of intramuscular pressure, Surgery **79**:702, 1976.
32. Mavor, G.E.: The anterior tibial syndrome, J. Bone Joint Surg. **38B**:513, 1956.
33. Mozes, M., Ramon, Y., and Jahr, J.: The anterior tibial syndrome, J. Bone Joint Surg. **44A**:730, 1962.
34. Mubarak, S.J., and Owen, C.A.: Double incision fasciotomy of the leg for decompression in compartment syndromes, J. Bone Joint Surg. **59A**:184, 1977.
35. Mubarak, S.J., and Hargens, A.R.: Exertional compartment syndromes. In Mubarak, S.J., and others: Compartment syndromes and Volkmann's contracture, Philadelphia, 1981, W.B. Saunders Co.
36. Mubarak, S.J., and others: The wick catheter technique for measurement of intramuscular pressure: a new research and clinical tool, J. Bone Joint Surg. **58A**:1016, 1976.
37. Mubarak, S.J., and others: Acute compartment syndromes: diagnosis and treatment with the aid of the wick catheter, J. Bone Joint Surg. **60A**:1091, 1978.
38. Mubarak, S.J., and others: Acute exertional superficial posterior compartment syndrome, Am. J. Sports Med. **6**:287, 1978.
39. Owen, C.A., and others: Intramuscular fluid pressure during isometric contraction, unpublished paper, 1981.
40. Paton, D.F.: The pathogenesis of anterior tibial syndrome, J. Bone Joint Surg. **50B**:383, 1968.
41. Pearson, C., Adams, R.D., and Denny-Brown, D.: Traumatic necrosis of pretibial muscles, N. Engl. J. Med. **231**:213, 1948.
42. Puranen, J.: The medial tibial syndrome: exercise ischemia in the medial fascial compartment of the leg, J. Bone Joint Surg. **56B**:712, 1974.
43. Reid, R.L., and Travis, R.T.: Acute necrosis of the second interosseous compartment of the hand, J. Bone Joint Surg. **55A**:1095, 1973.
44. Reneman, R.S.: The anterior and the lateral compartment syndrome of the leg, The Hague, 1968, Mouton Co.
45. Reneman, R.S.: The anterior and the lateral compartmental syndrome of the leg due to intensive use of muscles, Clin. Orthop. **113**:69, 1975.
46. Rorabeck, C.H.: Personal communication, 1981.
47. Rorabeck, C.H., and others: Compartmental pressure measurements: an experimental investigation using the slit catheter, J. Trauma **21**:446, 1981.
48. Rosato, F.E., and others: Subcutaneous fasciotomy: description of a new technique and instrument, Surgery **59**:383, 1966.
49. Sirbu, A.B., Murphy, M.J., and White, A.S.: Soft tissue complications of fracture of the leg, Cal. West. Med. **60**:53, 1944.
50. Slocum, D.B.: The shin splint syndrome: medical aspects and differential diagnosis, Am. J. Surg. **114**:875, 1967.
51. Snook, G.A.: Intermittent claudication in athletes, J. Sports Med. **3**:71, 1975.
52. Tompkins, D.G.: Exercise myopathy of the extensor carpi ulnaris muscle: report of a case, J. Bone Joint Surg. **59A**:407, 1977.
53. Veith, R.G., Matsen, F.A., III, and Newell, S.G.: Recurrent anterior compartmental syndromes, Phys. Sportsmed. **8**:80, 1980.
54. Vogt, P.R.: Ischemic muscular necrosis following marching, Oregon State Med. Soc., September 4, 1943 (cited in ref. 23).
55. Wells, H.S., Youmans, J.B., and Miller, D.G., Jr.: Tissue pressure (intracutaneous, subcutaneous, and intramuscular) as related to venous pressure, capillary filtration, and other factors, J. Clin. Invest. **17**:489, 1938.
56. Whitesides, T.E., Jr., and others: Tissue pressure measurements as a determinant for the need of fasciotomy, Clin. Orthop. **113**:43, 1975.
57. Wolfort, F.G., Mogelvang L.C., and Filtzer, H.S.: Anterior tibial compartment syndrome following muscle hernia repair, Arch. Surg. **106**:97, 1973.
58. Wright, S.: Applied physiology, ed. 10, London, 1961, Oxford University Press.

18. Overall view of rehabilitation of the leg for running

Robert E. Leach

Before I make some general comments on rehabilitation, let me give one basic precept. Not all injured athletes and certainly not all injured runners will be able to return to their preinjury status. Some—one hopes only a few—will no longer be able to perform at competitive level. There is no law stating that the final result is a return to competitive running or that each runner will be able to set increasingly long distances as his personal record. Runners seem to be highly motivated, and in that motivation is an almost neurotic compulsion to push themselves farther and farther. As physicians, we must try to set realistic goals.

If a runner has an injury to a structure in the leg, the rehabilitation program must pay particular attention to the injured area. However, in our haste to deal with a specific injury, we must not forget to deal with the whole lower extremity. For instance, a runner with a chronic knee problem will also have weakness and atrophy of the muscles around the hip and calf. We cannot rehabilitate only the muscles that control the knee.

There are four basic requirements to which rehabilitation therapy should be directed: range of motion, strength, endurance, and proprioception.

The patient must regain a normal range of motion of all joints of the lower extremity—the hip, knee, ankle, and subtalar joint—to function optimally while running. Although the hip and the knee are easy joints to rehabilitate, it may be hard to regain total passive dorsiflexion and normal inversion and eversion of the foot. Thus a runner placed in a cast for a period of time for a fracture of the tibia or a knee injury may find after the cast is removed that restoration of passive foot dorsiflexion and subtalar motion is the major long-term problem. The therapist must stay within the limits of the athlete's pain, or early gains will be lost.

After the range of motion comes back, athletes usually develop muscle strength next. This is done by providing resistance to muscle groups. If the knee has been injured, it is easy to work on the quadriceps or hamstrings because rehabilitation equipment is widely available for these muscles. However, for total lower extremity rehabilitation, therapy must also include the hip flexors, extensors, abductors, and adductors and the dorsiflexors and plantar flexors of the foot. It is harder to work on the muscles of the lower leg and the hip. I sometimes ask patients to tie one end of a piece of surgical tubing to a fixed point and the other end around the leg. They work against the resistance of the surgical tubing to improve foot inversion, eversion, and dorsiflexion.

When they begin to find their strength approaching a normal level, most athletes believe they are ready to return to complete activity. Sometimes, although they feel good at first, their endurance is below par and their performance suffers after a short period of athletic activity. Endurance takes much longer than strength to return; repetitive exercises and weight resistance are necessary to gradually rebuild muscle bulk. Most athletes do not regain their normal endurance until they have overcome the muscle atrophy previously sustained. This may take 6 to 12 months even in highly trained athletes. Some athletes improve both strength and endurance by working with high weights and fewer repetitions on one day and switching to lower weights and more repetitions the next day.

Proprioception is the athlete's ability to know where his body is in relation to space and to other objects around him. This sense disappears easily after an injury or surgery.[1] Sometimes it disappears simply when the athlete is away from his sport. Many times an athlete comes back from an injury having regained range of motion, strength, and even endurance and yet does not perform well. I believe that the proprioceptive sense is less easily restored than the other functions. During the rehabilitative process I give athletes a number of drills and agility tests to help them regain their proprioceptive sense in preparation for a return to such skills as hurdling, running, and pole vaulting.

One final comment on rehabilitation and proprioception: rehabilitation should be started with treatment and not at the end of treatment. The longer the athlete is withheld from his sport or from beginning his rehabilitation, the more he loses his sense of proprioception. Runners and other track athletes must begin exercise as soon after an injury as possible. The use of cast braces, transcutaneous electrical neural stimulation, cold, and other physical modalities that enable athletes to begin working more quickly is important. This prevents a long-term dissociation from their normal proprioception, and they will return to action more quickly and at a higher level.

REFERENCE

1. Freeman, M.A.R., and Wybe, B.: Articular contributions to limb muscle reflexes: the effects of partial neurectomy of the knee joint on postural reflexes, Br. J. Surg. **53**:61, 1966.

19. Return to running after injury

William J. Bowerman

CASE 1

Patient: Henry Marsh

Event: Steeplechase (3000 m, 27 hurdles, 7 water jumps)

Problem: Enlarged synovial band resulting from overwork

Treatment (by Dr. Stanley James, orthopedic surgeon): Snipping

Henry Marsh was a pleasant man to train. He had been in an outstanding track program coached by Clarence Robison at Brigham Young University. Marsh's intelligence and logic bore the mark of his personal religious philosophy and his educational pursuit as a third-year law student at the University of Oregon. His overwork from September to November 1979 led to his physical breakdown and subsequent successful treatment by Dr. James. As a result of Marsh's dedication to his physician's guidance and the total cooperation of athlete, physician, and coach, he broke the U.S. record for the steeplechase by 5 seconds in the 1980 Olympic trials.

The following is the rehabilitation program that Dr. James prescribed for Marsh before his return to a full training schedule. I am very much in agreement with Dr. James' underwork procedure, and I believe that Marsh's recovery illustrates its benefits.

  1. *Walking* after warm-up and stretching
      First week (Mon., Wed., Fri., Sat.)
          100 yards slow
          100 yards fast
          8 laps a day
      Second week (Mon., Wed., Fri., Sat.)
          200 yards fast
          200 yards slow
          12 laps a day

2. *Running* after warm-up and stretching
    Third week (Mon., Wed., Fri.)
        Alternate 15 minutes slow
                20 minutes medium
    Fourth week (Mon., Wed., Fri.)
        Alternate 20 minutes slow
                25 minutes medium
    Fifth week (Mon., Wed., Fri.)
        Alternate 25 minutes slow
                30 minutes medium
    Sixth week (Mon.-Sat.)
        Alternate 30 minutes slow
                40 minutes medium
3. Return to normal training

Whenever possible I like to base an individual's training program on a test run. The athlete may choose to run 800 m ($^1/_2$ mile), 1 mile, or 3 miles. In the absence of other deciding factors, it is easiest to use the 800-m run for the test.

I ask the runner how fast he can run 800 m on that day.

He may reply, "Between 2:05 and 2:10."

"Fine," I say. "Let's make it a three-fourths maximum effort and run 68 to 70 seconds per lap. The first 200 meters must not be run faster than 34 seconds, and the last 200 can be at nine-tenths effort if you want."

I place a marker in the middle of each straight and the middle of each curve to mark 200 m or 220 yards. The test is started and finished in the middle of the straight.

In his test Marsh ran the first 220 yards in 34 seconds, the first lap in 67 seconds, and the first 220 yards of the second lap in 32 seconds. He finished comfortably with a total time of 2 minutes, 8 seconds. Obviously, had he run each lap in 61 seconds, his time would have been 2 minutes, 2 seconds. But I believe that in practice, as in competition, a race should be started slowly and finished fast. I want the athletes I coach to run in practice as they would in a race.

Having established a three-fourths effort pace for 800 m of 65 seconds per lap, I made the following calculations. At three-fourths effort the runner could run 1 mile at 70 seconds per lap, 3000 m or 2 miles at 75 seconds per lap, and 5000 m at 80 seconds per lap. Therefore, based on my experience and arbitrary estimate, I established the date pace at full effort:

Distance	Three-fourths effort pace	Date pace
800 m	68-70 seconds per lap	60-65 seconds per lap
1 mile	73-75 seconds per lap	65-70 seconds per lap
Steeplechase (3000 m)	78-80 seconds per lap	70-75 seconds per lap

Using these figures, I made a graph for Marsh that included the 800 m, 1 mile, and steeplechase and progressed from the start of training in February to the Olympic trials in June.

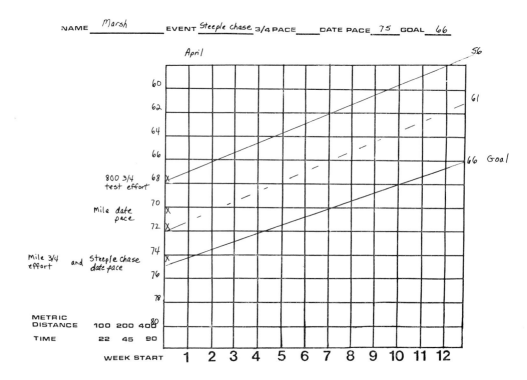

Prescription for training

After his 6 weeks of therapy training, the following prescription or pattern of training was developed for Marsh on the basis of his test run:

Jog in the early morning when convenient. Afternoon workouts are as follows:

MON.: Long run (8 to 10 miles) at 6 to 8 minutes per mile

TUES.: Light day or intervals: 1 × 3 laps over jumps at 75 seconds per lap
                                    2 × 2 laps at 73 seconds, second lap over jumps
                                    2 × 1 lap at 71 seconds, second 220 over jumps
                                    2 × 200 flat at seven-eighths effort
                                    (total distance 2½ miles, recovery
                                    pulse down to 120 before next interval)

WED.: Easy day: swim, lift weights, or jog 30 minutes at a pace of 8-10 minutes per mile

THURS.: Intervals of one-half racing distance—600 m at date pace, 400 m at 1 to 2 seconds less than date pace, 200 m at seven-eighths effort
Fartlek run

FRI.: Swim or jog 30 minutes

SAT.: Run a simulated race (1 mile, steeplechase, or 2 miles) at three-fourths effort

SUN.: Meditation and time with family

CASE 2

Patient: Jon Anderson

Event: 10,000 m (U.S. Olympic Team, 1972; All American, 1973), marathon (Boston Marathon winner, 1973)

Problem: Pump-bump syndrome, gradual running disability

Treatment (by Dr. Stanley James, orthopedic surgeon): Decompression

After Anderson's operation, Dr. James recommended a rehabilitation program similar to that prescribed for Henry Marsh. Over a period of about 6 weeks Anderson progressed from walking to easy running over gradually increasing distances. When Anderson, Dr. James, and I, the consulting coach, agreed that he was ready, he began using a typical schedule for marathon training.

The training schedule should be used as a guide, not a mandate, and should be continually assessed and revised to suit the individual's ability and progress. Overwork evidenced by undue fatigue or injury should be avoided.

The purposes of the exercises used in marathon training are the following:

1. To learn pace judgment
2. To accomplish the physical "tune-up" required to cover the distance
3. To learn and practice the strategies of the marathon race
4. To conform to the "hard-easy" principle that allows the body to recover between heavy workouts (a principle called the "Oregon system" by *Track and Field News* because it has worked well at the University of Oregon through many successful years)
5. To try a variety of exercises that have worked for other athletes, eliminating those that do not seem to contribute to the individual's expected progress

Prescription for marathon training

The following pattern for marathon training is similar to that used by Anderson while I served as his consulting coach. After his operation and rehabilitation program, this training prescription brought him to a new level of competitive fitness for the Nike Marathon in Eugene, Oregon, in September 1980. In that race he improved his previous best time (at the Boston Marathon) by nearly 5 minutes, completing the race in 2 hours, 12 minutes.

First 3 weeks

FIRST SUN.:	Run 10 to 12 miles at half effort (8, 10, or 12 minutes per mile)
MON.:	Light exercise
TUES.:	1. Intervals (1 mile or $^3/_4$ mile repeated three to six times at marathon racing pace with recovery between each)
	2. Fartlek (varied pace running including sprints and race tactics with recovery periods of easy jogging)
	3. Finish on the grass with slow, medium, and fast 100-m runs
WED.:	Light day—swimming or weight-lifting and 20-minute jog

THURS.: Steady-state run for 45 minutes to $1^1/2$ hours at half to three-fourths effort (6 to 8 minutes per mile), followed by 110-m runs on the grass

FRI.: Light exercise

SAT.: Road race or fartlek

SECOND SUN.: Run 14 to 16 miles at half effort

THIRD SUN.: Run 15 to 18 miles at half effort

This 3-week pattern is repeated with the distance of the Sunday runs differing. The maximum mileage of 27 to 30 miles at half effort is probably run on the ninth Sunday of training.

Second 3 weeks

FOURTH SUN.: Run 10 to 12 miles

FIFTH SUN.: Run 10 to 12 miles

SIXTH SUN.: Run 20 to 25 miles (plenty of liquids)

Third 3 weeks

SEVENTH SUN.: Run 10 to 12 miles

EIGHTH SUN.: Run 10 to 12 miles

NINTH SUN.: Run 25 to 30 miles (plenty of liquids)

REMINDER: Any schedule such as that above is intended as a *guide* and should be adapted by the athlete, coach, or physician according to the runner's ability and progress.

20. A running psychologist speaks of running

Bruce C. Ogilvie

As the costs of physical and emotional care have escalated during the last decade, more health professionals have become advocates of personal health maintenance as the only viable solution. It has been estimated that approximately 27 million North Americans have turned to running as their major health maintenance exercise. Most investigators have separated these exercise enthusiasts into three levels of personal commitment: the novice who averages between 3 and 6 miles a week, the more committed runner who averages between 12 and 16 miles a week, and the competitive runner who averages more than 30 miles a week. This distinction has been important because psychological differences and physical problems have been found to be related to the intensity, frequency, and duration of running. Any health prescription program that does not inform the beginning runner of the physical and emotional dangers inherent in this form of fitness would be professionally irresponsible.

This warning should need little reinforcement because running for health maintenance is continually having to be defended in the face of media attacks or the presentation of sensationalized case histories. It is entirely possible by the use of homogeneous samples and selected cases to present an argument that running may negatively effect psychological, social, and physical health. Two excellent examples are the articles by Morgan[13-15] and Peele.[17]

Shipman[18] in her article in *The Runner* presents convincing data from her survey of 250 runners that personality and values struggles may produce a variety of marital conflicts. It is too soon to attribute these conflicts directly to the desire to run, but it is clear that exercise addiction can exacerbate already existing personal conflicts. Shipman's evidence is consistent with Kostrubala's generalization that "running has profound effects on personal relationships."[11]

Johnson[10] provides evidence to support the point of view of anyone who chooses a sedentary life-style. He begins by stating, "In pursuit of an elusive feeling of well-being—even invincibility—some runners may actually have turned into addicts, and the monkey on their backs is wearing jogging shoes."[10] By his selective use of the published works of Glasser, Sacks, Morgan,[13] Peele, Bittker, and Gerwitz he is able to document the extremes to which some individuals go in their quest for physical health.

That exercise addiction may be a danger for those who make systematic running an important part of their lives should not be unexpected. The threat of addiction is inherent in any activity in which the individual seeks some form of ego satisfaction.

THE CASE FOR RUNNING AS A MENTAL HEALTH ACTIVITY

It is rarely possible when researching the literature to find almost universally positive empirical support for a human activity. With respect to the relationship between running and emotional health, however, the findings are universally supportive with the exception of concern for exercise addiction.

The investigations in the early 1970s by Ismail and Young[8] and Heinzelmann and Bagley[7a] were the first of a number of studies designed to determine the psychological effects of physical activities.[9] These researchers and all subsequent investigators have reported that systematic exercise programs significantly improve the emotional state of the participant and profoundly affect basic attitudes.

In his earlier investigations Ismail's subjects were patients who had undergone a cardiac event. They were separated into sedentary control and exercise groups. After 3 months the experimental subjects in the exercise group measured significantly higher for those factors associated with emotional health and self-esteem. They expressed an increased exuberance for life and looked forward more positively to the future.

The Heinzelmann Three-University Pilot Study[7a] was designed to determine if high-risk men placed in a program of physical activity would differ from like men in a control sedentary group. In comparison with the sedentary controls, the physically active men reported less stress and tension, feelings of better health, and increased stamina.

The other life-style changes in the physically active men may have even greater significance for those involved in the promotion of health maintenance principles, since these changes suggest a profound alteration in attitudes and values. The physically active group lost more weight, slept better, and reported a sense of increased work performance accompanied by a more positive reaction to work. There is a growing body of evidence that physical activity, particularly aerobic exercise, greatly improves the quality of the individual's life-style.

Ismail, Corrigan, and Young[9] have recently completed a study that may do more to promote an increased financial investment in health maintenance than all the foregoing findings combined. This study was designed to examine the effects of regular exercise on life-style by comparing the frequency and dollar amount of nonaccident medical insurance claims for exercising and sedentary subjects over a 4-year period. The study found that the exercising group had significantly fewer and lower dollar amount insurance claims than the nonexercising group. At the end of the study the subjects exercising regularly had lower body weight, lower resting heart rate, lower diastolic blood pressure, and lower submaximal heart rate. They also had a higher percentage of lean body mass and a greater maximum oxygen uptake. Once again the high fitness scores for the exercise group correlated with healthier personality characteristics, particularly those related to emotional stability.

The psychological findings of Ismail, Corrigan, and Young[9] are pertinent to the central concern of this chapter, the relationship between exercise and mental health. They reported that at the termination of the study the exercise group was emotionally more stable, experienced greater inner peace, and was more insightful. They also possessed greater self-control and functioned at a lower level of body tension. Thus "the exercising group tended to have a more desirable psychological profile than the non-exercising group; particularly in the direction of increased emotional stability."[9]

This longitudinal study is valuable because it supports the findings of past investigations studying exercise programs of much shorter duration, but the medical cost data reported may have the most profound influence. During the 4-year period of the study, the average yearly medical costs for the nonexercise group were more than double those of the exercisers, or $390.53 as compared with $166.41.

RUNNING AS A MIND-ALTERING EXPERIENCE

Since the mid-1960s there has been an increased use of running as a treatment for depression. Greist and co-workers,[7] in a review of the literature and of their own research at the University of Wisconsin Outpatient Clinic, concluded that running is a reliable treatment for depression. They reported that six of their eight mentally depressed patients who ran for 30 to 45 minutes three times a week were "essentially well within three weeks and remained well for the duration of active treatment." They found that "running can literally cure some moderate depressions, and it may reduce anxiety, and in many patients can replace antidepressants."[7]

The International Association of Running Therapists was organized by Kostrubala in 1980 as an outgrowth of his personal experience with running as a therapeutic technique.[12] Through running he reduced his cardiovascular risk factors and lost his symptoms of depression. He also developed increased ego strength and was able to reorganize his personality.

The mind-altering potential of running, exercise, and sport is receiving serious attention. Murphy and White[16] have documented at least 30 types of mental experiences that have been reported by athletes to have had a profound effect upon their consciousness. These mental experiences ranged from spiritual healing to psychokinesis and even immunity to harm. Whether such experiences lead to a significant alteration in values, personality, or life-style must await future research.

RUNNING AS A FORM OF ADDICTION

Morgan[14] and co-workers[15] present an excellent case as to the potential negative effects that can be produced socially, psychologically, and physically when one becomes a "running addict." Morgan defines the hard-core exercise addict as a person who "can't live without daily running, manifests withdrawal symptoms if deprived of exercise, and runs even when his physician says he shouldn't."[15] According to Bittker,

> We may begin running just to stay in shape but soon are seduced by the sense of clarity, energy and self-esteem accompanying the daily run. Having achieved reasonable conditioning, we run farther and faster in an attempt to find our peak. It is at this point that our tragic flaw emerges. Our gluttony may once again conquer us.[1]

Advocates of running for emotional and physical health should counsel the novice runner as to the mental health approach to fitness. Beginners should learn to recognize the symptoms of running addiction and should direct their behavior toward a rational commitment to this activity.

The major symptom is the psychological withdrawal that may occur when the runner is forced to reduce his running or stop for a week or more. Any restriction of the runner's habitual routine results in anxiety, tension, or extreme irritability. The anxiety may take the form of a depression supported by deep feelings of guilt. Muscle tension, loss of sleep, decreased appetite, and constipation are often reported.

The emotional confusion generated by addiction to running is not limited to personal idiosyncracies but spills over into social, marital, and even career areas. When the need to run takes priority over family, friends, job, or intimate interaction with others, professional intervention may be the only reasonable course of action.

The evidence that the runner has become addicted may be first observed during the medical examination for an overuse syndrome. Many case histories have described extremes of irrational behavior in regard to runners' pain tolerance and denial. These exercise addicts have been willing to subject themselves to any form of treatment, injection, or mechanical device that will permit them to seek their "fix." The following two case histories are of individuals who have recently sought my counsel.

CASE 1

A 47-year-old professional man was preparing for a California ultramarathon (100 miles). His running program was designed to cover an average of 90 miles a week. He was about five feet seven inches tall and weighed about 120 pounds.

He asked me to teach him some psychological technique that would enable him to manage the pain and discomfort he felt during training. His painful symptom was medical in nature and he was being treated by a qualified specialist. He was determined to continue to train with one of the worst cases of ruptured hemorrhoids that I have ever heard described. He spent considerable time designing sanitary napkins that would enable him to keep up his training. He was ready to try salves, ointments, belts, straps, or any conceivable aid so that he would be able to compete in the ultramarathon. He found my reluctance to become a party to his masochistic quest both offensive and unprofessional.

CASE 2

A 42-year-old marathon runner consulted me after having failed to complete a 100-mile ultramarathon. He presented the classic clinical picture of an agitated depressive reaction.

His case is relevant because it shows the extent to which the irrationality of the addicted runner may be carried. Whatever meaning this patient's fitness program might have had originally was now tangled within a subconscious form of self-destruction.

At some point in the forty-seventh mile he sustained a serious ankle injury that necessitated medical team support to get him down off the trail. He seemed almost delighted that it had been an injury that had taken him out of competition. It was of paramount importance to him that he was transported down under medical care so that all the world could see he was not a quitter. He continually mentioned that the injury had enabled him to salvage his self-respect so he could now live with himself.

In this patient a basically healthy activity had become perverted to serve his neurotic needs. It was evident that he was attempting to use running as a means of proving something about himself as a person that could never be attained through success in this activity.

PSYCHOLOGICAL PREPARATION OF THE FEMALE RUNNER

Cooper[2] has stated that in 1968 there were about 100,000 runners but that by 1979 the figures were as high as 17 million. Certainly those of us who run for health are becoming aware of the increasing number of female runners. Although a vast literature exists concerning the physiological differences between men and women, studies of psychological differences are extremely limited in number.

Investigations of the effects of running on the female menstrual cycle have been of inestimable value because of the possible psychological implications for competitive women runners.[19] The published research has enabled women to become better educated about the endocrinological facts of life, and this information is useful to relieve unnecessary anxiety. Medical research has also provided helpful information concerning the effects of running on the female breast. Such information has done much to destroy old myths and provide psychological comfort for the female athlete.

It is important for health professionals to be aware of the higher incidence of injury in novice female runners. Gendel,[4] in her article dealing with lack of fitness as a contributing factor in chronic illness in women, reviewed the psychosocial factors that have kept women from becoming as exercise conscious as men.

Franklyn, Lussier, and Buskirk[3] found that jogging-related injury rates for male novices ranged up to 54% and were related to the intensity, frequency, and duration of training. The injury rate for the beginning female joggers was 82% by the end of the first 6 weeks of training. These were minor injuries, mostly joint sprains, muscle strains, shin splints, and foot ailments.

Gottlieb and White[6] recently reported an incidence of injury of 86% for recreational runners, and Glick and Katch[5] in 1970 gave a figure of 90%. A questionnaire sent out by *Runner's World* found a significant correlation between injury rate and miles run per week. Of those running more than 50 miles per week, 73% reported injuries, while 34% of those running less than 25 miles per week had had an injury.

The threat of injury, discomfort, and pain may play an important role in discouraging women from taking up running. Since only 10% of beginning runners will have no physical discomfort, the health professional must prescribe a running program wisely to reduce the incidence of early injury and help the runner to remain motivated should some mild injury occur. As previously mentioned, there is a high correlation between injury and intensity, frequency, and duration of exercise. We must counter the prevailing philosophy that "more is better" or that one "must hurt to improve" and teach novices to pay attention to their bodies.

Our responsibility to the female runner is much greater than to the male because the sedentary woman who takes up running will face more intense emotional and physical adaptation stresses. She may have doubts as to the appropriateness of her becoming a dedicated athlete. Therefore she must receive more attention and an empathic concern with regard to her psychological and physical preparation. It takes between 6 and 12 weeks of training before the runner begins to experience the intrinsic rewards. Our goal should be to provide guidance so that each novice reaches this point of conditioning.

RUNNING AND MARITAL HARMONY

Although a single study of 250 individuals such as that reported by Shipman[18] does not permit many generalizations, it suggests that running can be hazardous to marital relationships. Her respondents confirmed early research that personality, values, and life-styles may change dramatically. According to Shipman,

First runners experience an almost immediate increase in self confidence as a result of their improved physical condition. They soon discover more energy to invest in their work and creative projects. Eventually they tend to shed their non-running friends and develop new and stronger bonds with other runners, based upon shared commitments to diet and nutrition, to keep regular hours and to spend more time out of doors.[18]

These life-style changes can impose new stresses on an already strained relationship.

Shipman found that the male runner and his nonrunning wife had only a 50% chance of working out problems in their relationship. The relationship at greatest hazard was that of the running woman married to a sedentary husband. Running women reported that they began to find their mates less than satisfying. Male runners, however, believed that running enhanced their marital relationships whether or not their wives were runners.

Shipman reported that the frequency of sexual intercourse dropped for all runners, both male and female, while the quality of sexual experience improved. The highest level of sexual compatibility was found when both partners were runners.

She concluded that running is a catalyst bringing conflicts to the surface rather than an underlying cause of divorce and separation. Her study supports the consistently reported finding that a commitment to running contributes to a profound alteration in personality, life-style, and values.

REFERENCES

1. Bittker, T.: Running gluttony, Runner's World **12**:10, 1977.
2. Cooper, K.: Runner's World exclusive, Runner's World **14**:26, 1979.
3. Franklyn, B., Lussier, L., and Buskirk, E.: Injury rates in women joggers, Phys. Sportsmed. **8**:42, 1980.
4. Gendel, E.S.: Lack of fitness: a source of chronic ills in women, Phys. Sportsmed. **6**:85, 1978.

5. Glick, J.M., and Katch, V.L.: Musculoskeletal injuries in jogging, Arch. Phys. Med. Rehabil. **51:**123, 1970.
6. Gottlieb, G., and White, J.R.: Response of recreational runners to their injuries, Phys. Sportsmed. **8:**145, 1980.
7. Greist, J.H., and others: Running out of depression, Phys. Sportsmed. **6:**49, 1978.
8. Ismail, A.H., and Young, R.J.: The effects of chronic exercise on the personality of middle-aged men by univariate and multivariate approaches, J. Hum. Ergol. **2:**45, 1973.
9. Ismail, A.H., Corrigan, D.L., and Young, R.J.: The effects of habitual exercise on general health as reflected by nonaccident insurance claims, unpublished paper presented to U.S. Department of Health and Human Services, July 1980.
10. Johnson, W.D.: Marching to euphoria, Sports Illustrated **53:**18, 1980.
11. Kostrubala, T.: Prescription for stress: running, Practical Psychol. Phys. **2:**50, 1975.
12. Kostrubala, T.: Running therapy, Phys. Sportsmed. **8:**97, 1980.
13. Morgan, W.: Mind of the marathoner, Psychology Today **2:**38, 1978.
14. Morgan, W.: Negative addiction in runners, Phys. Sportsmed. **7:**57, 1979.
15. Morgan, W., Roberts, J., and Brant, F.: Psychological effects of chronic physical activity, Med. Science Sports **2:**213, 1970.
16. Murphy, M., and White, R.: The psychic side of sports, Reading, Mass., 1978, Addison-Wesley Publishing Co., Inc.
17. Peele, S.: Addiction—analgesic experience, Human Nature **1:**9, 1978.
18. Shipman, C.: Social cost of running, The Runner **3:**47, 1980.
19. Speroff, L., and Redwine, D.: Exercise and menstrual function, Phys. Sportsmed. **8:**42, 1980.

Index